Stahl's Illustrated

Anxiety, Stress, and PTSD

Stephen M. Stahl
University of California, San Diego

Meghan M. Grady
Neuroscience Education Institute

Nancy Muntner
Illustrations

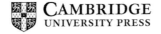

CAMBRIDGE
UNIVERSITY PRESS

CAMBRIDGE UNIVERSITY PRESS
Cambridge, New York, Melbourne, Madrid, Cape Town, Singapore,
São Paulo, Delhi, Dubai, Tokyo

Cambridge University Press
32 Avenue of the Americas, New York, NY 10013-2473, USA

www.cambridge.org
Information on this title: www.cambridge.org/9780521153997

© Neuroscience Education Institute 2010

First published 2010

Printed in the United States of America

A catalog record for this publication is available from the British Library.

Library of Congress Cataloging in Publication data
Stahl, S. M.
Anxiety, stress, and PTSD / Stephen M. Stahl, Nancy Muntner ; illustrations, Meghan M. Grady.
   p. ; cm. – (Stahl's illustrated series)
Includes bibliographical references and index.
ISBN 978-0-521-15399-7 (pbk.)
1. Post-traumatic stress disorder – Treatment – Handbooks, manuals, etc.   2. Anxiety –
Chemotherapy – Handbooks, manuals, etc.   I. Muntner, Nancy.   II. Neuroscience Education Institute.
III. Title.   IV. Series: Stahl's illustrated series.
[DNLM: 1. Anxiety Disorders – drug therapy – Handbooks.   2. Anti-Anxiety Agents – pharmacology –
Handbooks.   3. Stress, Psychological – drug therapy – Handbooks. WM 34 S781a 2010]
RC552.P67S73   2010
616.85'21–dc22   2010012040

ISBN 978-0-521-15399-7 Paperback

Additional resources for this publication at www.neiglobal.com

Cambridge University Press has no responsibility for the
persistence or accuracy of URLs for external or third-party Internet
websites referred to in this publication and does not guarantee that
any content on such websites is, or will remain, accurate or
appropriate.

PREFACE

These books are designed to be fun, with all concepts illustrated by full-color images and the text serving as a supplement to figures, images, and tables. The visual learner will find that this book makes psychopharmacology concepts easy to master, while the non-visual learner may enjoy a shortened text version of complex psychopharmacology concepts. Each chapter builds upon previous chapters, synthesizing information from basic biology and diagnostics to building treatment plans and dealing with complications and comorbidities.

Novices may want to approach this book by first looking through all the graphics, gaining a feel for the visual vocabulary on which our psychopharmacology concepts rely. After this once-over glance, we suggest going back through the book to incorporate the images with supporting text. Learning from visual concepts and textual supplements should reinforce one another, providing you with solid conceptual understanding at each step along the way.

Readers more familiar with these topics should find that going back and forth between images and text provides an interaction with which to vividly conceptualize complex psychopharmacology. You may find yourself using this book frequently to refresh your psychopharmacological knowledge. And you will hopefully refer your colleagues to this desk reference.

This book is intended as a conceptual overview of different topics; we provide you with a visual-based language to incorporate the rules of psychopharmacology at the sacrifice of discussing the exceptions to these rules. A Suggested Readings section at the end gives you a good start for more in-depth learning about particular concepts presented here.

When you come across an abbreviation you don't understand, you can refer to the Abbreviations list in the back. *Stahl's Essential Psychopharmacology, 3rd Edition*, and *Stahl's Essential Psychopharmacology: The Prescriber's Guide, 3rd Edition*, can be helpful supplementary tools for more in-depth information on particular topics in this book. Now you can also search topics in psychopharmacology on the Neuroscience Education Institute's website (www.neiglobal.com) for lectures, courses, slides, and related articles.

Whether you are a novice or an experienced psychopharmacologist, hopefully this book will lead you to think critically about the complexities involved in psychiatric disorders and their treatments.

Best wishes for your educational journey into the fascinating field of psychopharmacology!

Stephen M. Stahl

Contents

CME Information

Overview
This book provides an overview of the latest developments in research and clinical treatment of posttraumatic stress disorder (PTSD). Chapter 1 covers the neurobiology of normal fear and worry and how genetic and environmental factors may interact to affect these circuits and increase risk for psychiatric illnesses such as PTSD. Chapter 2 covers the clinical presentation of PTSD, including comorbidities and suicidality as well as its underlying risk factors and neurobiology. Chapter 3 reviews the major neurotransmitter systems that regulate functioning within anxiety-related brain circuits, and that are therefore potential targets of pharmacologic action in the treatment of PTSD. Chapter 4 reviews the mechanisms of action and clinical characteristics of first-line pharmacologic treatments for PTSD, while Chapter 5 does the same for second-line, adjunct, and investigational agents, and Chapter 6 explains the methods for several first- and second-line cognitive behavioral therapies. Chapter 7 reviews diagnostic and treatment strategies for patients with PTSD, including consideration of comorbidities. Finally, Chapter 8 focuses on risks and complicating factors that are particularly relevant to the military population, with emphasis on the relationship between PTSD and the potential long-term effects of mild TBI.

Target Audience
This activity has been developed for prescribers specializing in psychiatry. There are no prerequisites for this activity. Health care providers in all specialties who are interested in psychopharmacology, especially primary care physicians, nurses, psychologists, and pharmacists, are welcome for advanced study.

Statement of Need
A surprisingly high percentage of the population will experience at least one traumatic event in their lifetime (trauma being defined as a frightening situation in which one experiences or witnesses the threat of death or injury). Although not all individuals exposed to traumatic events will develop psychopathology—in fact, most do not—a significant minority will, with potentially devastating consequences for them and their loved ones.

The following unmet needs regarding anxiety and posttraumatic stress disorder (PTSD) were revealed following a critical analysis of expert faculty assessment and literature review:

- PTSD is increasingly prevalent and associated with significant morbidity and mortality
- Neurobiology of stress and anxiety can serve to enhance understanding of anxious symptoms and their treatment
- Treatments for PTSD continue to be examined, with many options—both pharmacological and nonpharmacological—available based on individual symptoms

To help fill these unmet needs, quality improvement efforts need to provide education regarding (1) neurobiology of PTSD; (2) risk factors, both environmental and genetic, for PTSD; and (3) different therapeutic options available for PTSD and how to develop treatment strategies that maximize outcomes.

Learning Objectives
After completing this educational activity, participants should be better able to:

- Explain the neurobiology of both normal and pathological stress and anxiety
- Recognize the environmental and genetic factors that can contribute to the development of anxiety disorders
- Explain the pharmacology of therapeutic agents used in treating posttraumatic stress disorder (PTSD)
- Identify new drugs and methods in development for the treatment of PTSD
- Explain the principles and methods involved in cognitive behavioral therapy (CBT) for PTSD
- Customize treatment regimens for patients with PTSD based on symptom profile, comorbidities, and life situations

Accreditation and Credit Designation Statements

The Neuroscience Education Institute is accredited by the Accreditation Council for Continuing Medical Education to provide continuing medical education for physicians.

The Neuroscience Education Institute designates this educational activity for a maximum of 4.0 *AMA PRA Category 1 Credits™*. Physicians should only claim credit commensurate with the extent of their participation in the activity. Also available will be a certificate of participation for completing this activity.

Nurses may claim credit for activities approved for *AMA PRA Category 1 Credits™* in most states, for up to 50% of the nursing requirement for recertification. This activity is designated for 4.0 *AMA PRA Category 1 Credits*.

Activity Instructions

This CME activity is in the form of a printed monograph and incorporates instructional design to enhance your retention of the information and pharmacological concepts that are being presented. You are advised to go through the figures in this activity from beginning to end, followed by the text, and then complete the posttest and activity evaluation. The estimated time for completion of this activity is 4.0 hours.

Instructions for CME Credit

To receive your certificate of CME credit or participation, please complete the posttest (you must score at least 70% to receive credit) and activity evaluation found at the end of the monograph and mail or fax them to the address/number provided. Once received, your posttest will be graded and a certificate sent if a score of 70% or more was attained. Alternatively, **you may complete the posttest and activity evaluation online and immediately print your certificate.** There is a fee for the posttest (waived for NEI members).

NEI Disclosure Policy

It is the policy of the Neuroscience Education Institute to ensure balance, independence, objectivity, and scientific rigor in all its educational activities. Therefore, all individuals in a position to influence or control content development are required by NEI to disclose any financial relationships or apparent conflicts of interest that may have a direct bearing on the subject matter of the activity. Although potential conflicts of interest are identified and resolved prior to the activity being presented, it remains for the participant to determine whether outside interests reflect a possible bias in either the exposition or the conclusions presented.

These materials have been peer-reviewed to ensure the scientific accuracy and medical relevance of information presented and its independence from commercial bias. The Neuroscience Education Institute takes responsibility for the content, quality, and scientific integrity of this CME activity.

Individual Disclosure Statements
Authors
Meghan Grady
Director, Content Development, Neuroscience Education Institute, Carlsbad, CA
No other financial relationships to disclose.

Stephen M. Stahl, MD, PhD
Adjunct Professor, Department of Psychiatry, University of California, San Diego School of Medicine
Honorary Visiting Senior Fellow, University of Cambridge, UK
Grant/Research: Forest, Johnson & Johnson, Novartis, Organon, Pamlab, Pfizer, Sepracor, Shire, Takeda, Vanda, Wyeth
Consultant/Advisor: Arena, Azur, Bionevia, Boehringer Ingelheim, Bristol-Myers Squibb, CeNeRx, Dainippon Sumitomo, Eli Lilly, Endo, Forest, Janssen, Jazz, Johnson & Johnson, Labopharm, Lundbeck, Marinus, Neuronetics, Novartis, Noven, Pamlab, Pfizer, Pierre Fabre, Sanofi-Synthélabo, Sepracor, Servier, Shire, SK, Solvay, Somaxon, Tetragenix, Vanda
Speakers Bureau: Pfizer, Wyeth

Peer Reviewer
Ronnie Gorman Swift, MD
Professor and Associate Chairman, Department of Psychiatry and Behavioral Sciences, New York Medical College, Valhalla
Professor of Clinical Public Health, School of Public Health, New York; New York Medical College, Valhalla
Chief of Psychiatry and Associate Medical Director, Metropolitan Hospital Center, New York, NY
No other financial relationships to disclose.

Design Staff
Nancy Muntner
Director, Medical Illustrations, Neuroscience Education Institute, Carlsbad, CA
No other financial relationships to disclose.

Disclosed financial relationships have been reviewed by the Neuroscience Education Institute CME Advisory Board to resolve any potential conflicts of interest. All faculty and planning committee members have attested that their financial relationships do not affect their ability to present well-balanced, evidence-based content for this activity.

Disclosure of Off-Label Use

This educational activity may include discussion of products or devices that are not currently labeled for such use by the FDA. Please consult the product prescribing information for full disclosure of labeled uses.

Disclaimer

The information presented in this educational activity is not meant to define a standard of care, nor is it intended to dictate an exclusive course of patient management. Any procedures, medications, or other courses of diagnosis or treatment discussed or suggested in this educational activity should not be used by clinicians without full evaluation of their patients' conditions and possible contraindications or dangers in use, review of any applicable manufacturer's product information, and comparison with recommendations of other authorities. Primary references and full prescribing information should be consulted.

Participants have an implied responsibility to use the newly acquired information from this activity to enhance patient outcomes and their own professional development. The participant should use his/her clinical judgment, knowledge, experience, and diagnostic decision-making before applying any information, whether provided here or by others, for any professional use.

Sponsorship Information

This activity is sponsored by Neuroscience Education Institute.

Support

This activity is supported solely by the sponsor, Neuroscience Education Institute.
Neither the Neuroscience Education Institute nor the authors have received any funds or grants in support of this educational activity.

Date of Release/Expiration

Release Date: February 2010   CME Credit Expiration Date: January 2013

Stahl's Illustrated | Objectives

- Explain the neurobiology of both normal and pathological stress and anxiety

- Recognize the environmental and genetic factors that can contribute to the development of anxiety disorders

- Explain the pharmacology of therapeutic agents used in treating posttraumatic stress disorder (PTSD)

- Identify new drugs and methods in development for the treatment of PTSD

- Explain the principles and methods involved in cognitive behavioral therapy (CBT) for PTSD

- Customize treatment regimens for patients with PTSD based on symptom profile, comorbidities, and life situations

Neurobiology of Stress and Anxiety

Anxiety is a normal emotional and neurophysiological reaction to a perceived threat, and serves the purpose of preparing one to "freeze, take flight, or fight." Such a reaction is obviously an appropriate and even adaptive survival mechanism in the presence of actual threats, allowing one both to escape the current threat and to avoid future ones through conditioned fear learning. When the reaction occurs in the absence of a realistic threat, however—whether because the threat itself is unlikely or because harm from the perceived threat is unlikely—then it serves no useful purpose and instead can significantly disrupt one's ability to function, thus constituting an anxiety disorder.

There are several anxiety disorders, as defined in the *Diagnostic and Statistical Manual of Mental Disorders (DSM) IV-TR*, each with distinct characteristics, criteria, and symptoms, but all sharing the common core symptoms of excessive fear and worry. The neurobiological circuits underlying these core symptoms may thus be involved in all anxiety disorders, with the different phenotypes reflecting not unique circuitry but rather divergent malfunctioning within those circuits.

This chapter covers the neurobiology of normal fear and worry and how genetic and environmental factors may interact to affect these circuits and increase risk for psychiatric illnesses such as posttraumatic stress disorders (PTSD), which is the focus of this book.

SECTION ONE
The Core Symptoms of Anxiety Disorders: Fear and Worry

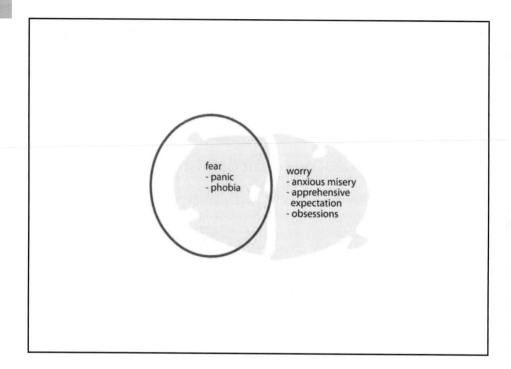

FIGURE 1.1. The two core symptoms shared by all anxiety disorders are anxiety or fear coupled with some form of worry. The circuitry mediating these two features is different, and will be addressed in turn, beginning with anxiety/fear.

The Amygdala's Role in Fear and Anxiety

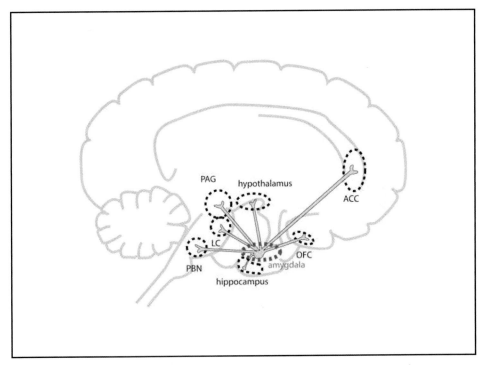

PAG: periaqueductal grey. LC: locus coeruleus. PBN: parabrachial nucleus.
OFC: orbitofrontal cortex. ACC: anterior cingulate cortex.

FIGURE 1.2. Anxiety is a state that encompasses both an internal "feeling" of fear and the physiological expression of that fear. Although separate circuits mediate these different aspects of anxiety, they share in common a central role of the amygdala, an almond-shaped limbic structure with widespread reciprocal connections with both higher and lower brain regions. As shown in Figures 1.3 through 1.9, the amygdala both regulates and is regulated by these other brain regions in order to produce (or suppress) a fear response.

Fear vs. Anxiety

TABLE 1.1.		
	DESCRIPTION	ANATOMICAL LOCALIZATION
fear	Short-term, stimulus-specific response	Basolateral, central, and medial nuclei of amygdala
anxiety	Sustained response influencing behavior after the stimulus is removed	Basolateral amygdala projections to bed nucleus of stria terminalis

The Amygdala and the Feeling of Fear

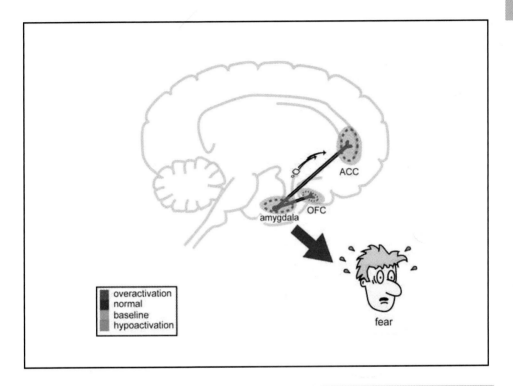

FIGURE 1.3. The emotional aspect of fear is regulated by connections between the amygdala and key areas of the prefrontal cortex, specifically the orbitofrontal cortex (OFC) and the anterior cingulate cortex (ACC).

The Amygdala and the Physiology of Fear:
Autonomic Output

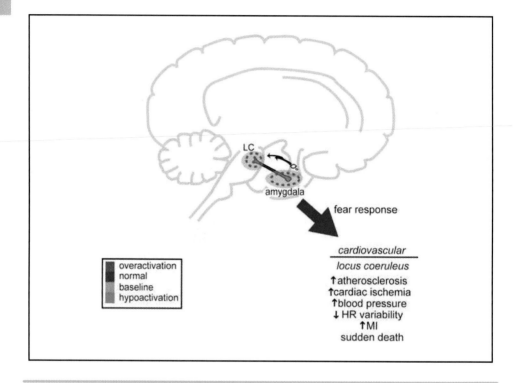

FIGURE 1.4. The physiological reaction to a fearful stimulus involves activation of multiple systems, including the autonomic system, as shown here. Activation of this system is regulated by connections between the amygdala and the locus coeruleus (LC), and leads to an increase in heart rate (HR) and blood pressure that is necessary for a fight/flight reaction.

Although acute activation of the autonomic nervous system is important for survival in response to real threats, chronic activation as part of an anxiety disorder can lead to increased risk of cardiovascular issues such as atherosclerosis, cardiac ischemia, hypertension, myocardial infarction (MI), or even sudden death.

The Amygdala and the Physiology of Fear:
Endocrine Output

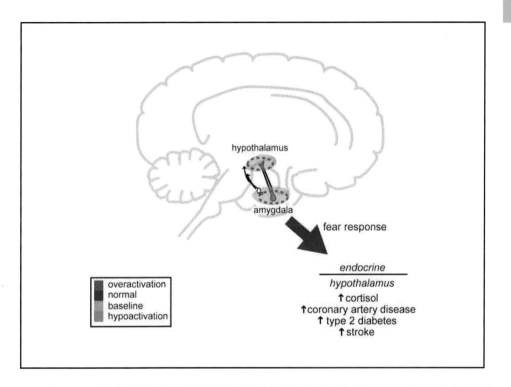

FIGURE 1.5. The hypothalamic pituitary adrenal (HPA) axis is responsible for endocrine output during the fear/stress response, and is regulated by the amygdala via reciprocal connections with the hypothalamus. During acute stress, such as exposure to a fearful stimulus, HPA activation increases the release of glucocorticoids such as cortisol, but only for a short time, until the perceived danger is gone. An abnormal stress response may occur due to chronic, unrelenting stress and/or due to stress during critical developmental periods, and can be associated with increased rates of medical complications such as coronary artery disease, type 2 diabetes, and stroke.

The role of the HPA axis in anxiety disorders is discussed in more detail in Figure 1.6 as well as in Figures 2.6 and 2.7.

The HPA Axis

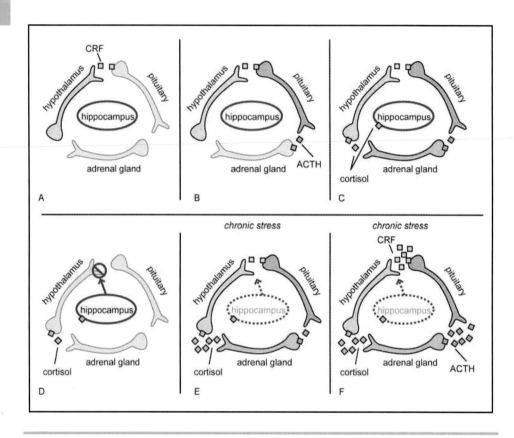

FIGURE 1.6. The central role of the HPA axis in stress processing makes it logical that it would be involved in the risk for anxiety disorders. The normal stress response involves activation of the hypothalamus and a resultant increase in corticotrophin releasing factor (CRF) (A), which in turn stimulates the release of adrenocorticotrophic hormone (ACTH) from the pituitary gland (B). ACTH causes glucocorticoid release (cortisol in humans) from the adrenal gland, which binds to receptors in the hypothalamus, pituitary, and hippocampus (C). Glucocorticoid binding in the hypothalamus inhibits CRF release, ending the stress response (D). In addition, the hippocampus plays a role in inhibiting the stress response (D).

In situations of chronic stress, excessive glucocorticoid release may eventually lead to hippocampal atrophy, thus preventing it from inhibiting the HPA axis (E). This could contribute to chronic activation of the HPA axis (F) and increase risk for an anxiety disorder.

The Amygdala and the Physiology of Fear:
Breathing Output

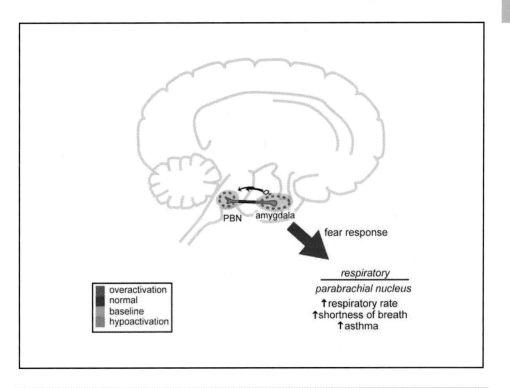

FIGURE 1.7. Increases in respiration rate are also an important part of a fear response and are regulated by connections between the amygdala and the parabrachial nucleus (PBN). However, when excessive activation occurs, this can cause shortness of breath, exacerbation of asthma, or a sense of being smothered—all of which are symptoms of a panic attack.

The Amygdala and the Behavior of Fear

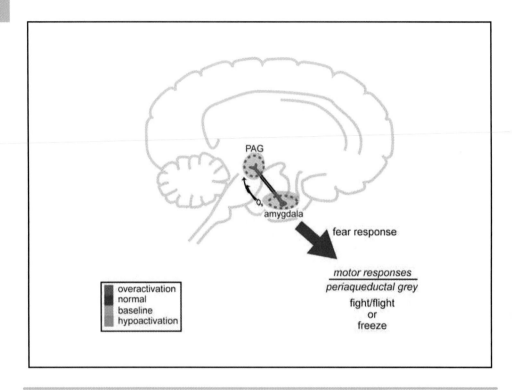

FIGURE 1.8. The emotional and physiological responses to a threat prepare one to take action in order to escape or combat that threat. The actual motor response taken—whether fight, flight, or freeze—is regulated in part through connections between the amygdala and the periaqueductal grey (PAG).

Stahl's Illustrated

The Hippocampus:
An Internal Fearmonger

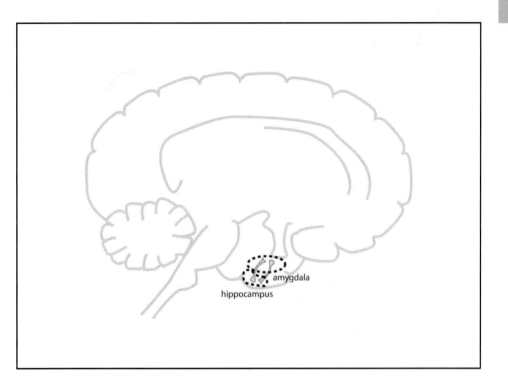

FIGURE 1.9. Anxiety can be triggered not only by an external stimulus but also internally through traumatic memories stored in the hippocampus, which can activate the amygdala and cause it, in turn, to activate other brain regions to generate a fear response. This is known as reexperiencing and is a central feature of posttraumatic stress disorder (PTSD).

Fear Conditioning

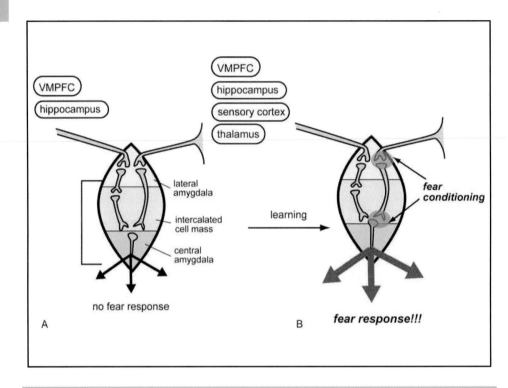

FIGURE 1.10. An important part of the normal fear response is the amygdala's ability to "remember" stimuli associated with the stressor so that it can react more efficiently if the stressor is ever reencountered—a process known as fear conditioning.

Upon acute exposure to a fearful situation, the lateral amygdala integrates input from several brain regions, including sensory cortex and thalamus, which provide information about stimuli associated with the fearful situation; the hippocampus, which provides memories of related fearful or traumatic experiences; and the ventromedial prefrontal cortex (VMPFC), which may provide mitigating input to suppress a fear response (A). If a fear response is in fact generated, then the amygdala restructures existing synapses to increase the efficiency of glutamatergic neurotransmission in response to future sensory input associated with the feared stimulus (B, represented by increased orange glutamate output and at synapses).

The Worry Loop

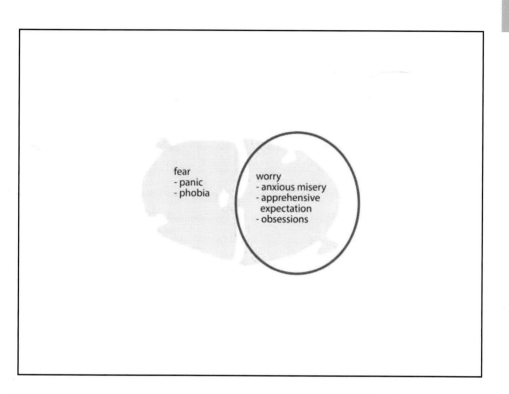

FIGURE 1.11. Figures 1.2 through 1.10 reviewed the circuitry of fear, one of the two core symptoms of all anxiety disorders. The second core symptom, worry, involves different circuitry, as shown in Figure 1.12.

Worry and Obsessions

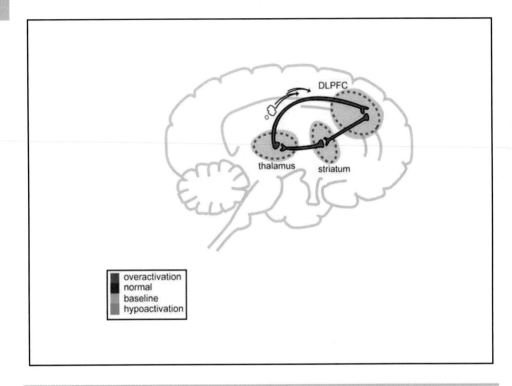

FIGURE 1.12. Worry, which can include apprehensive expectation, catastrophic thinking, and obsessions, is hypothetically linked to cortico-striatal-thalamic-cortical (CSTC) loops. Specifically shown here is a CSTC loop originating and ending in the dorsolateral prefrontal cortex (DLPFC).

SECTION TWO

The Path to Anxiety Disorders: A Circuit's Story

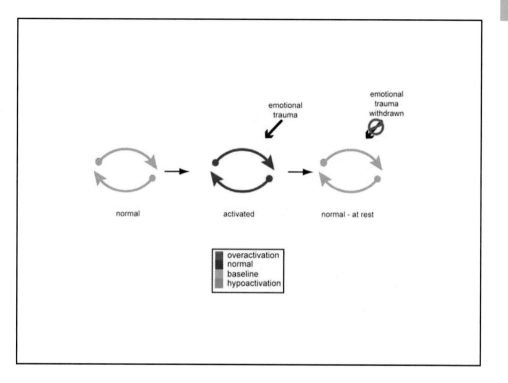

FIGURE 1.13. During acute exposure to stressors, the fear circuits described in Figures 1.3 through 1.9 are activated (middle), thus producing reactions that optimize the chances for survival. Once the trauma is withdrawn, the circuits return to baseline functioning (right). How then might activation of these circuits lead to the pathological symptoms of anxiety disorders?

Stress Sensitization in Normal Circuits

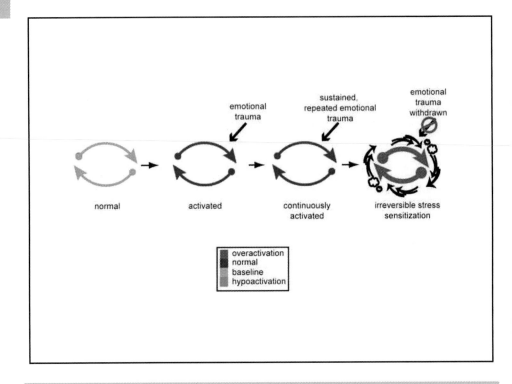

FIGURE 1.14. When circuits are repeatedly stressed and put on overload (middle right), it can lead to a condition known as "stress sensitization," in which circuits not only become overly activated but remain overly activated even when the stressor is withdrawn (right).

A sensitized circuit does not necessarily mean that symptoms will develop, however. Instead, overloading circuits can potentially result in a loss of resilience and development of vulnerability to future stressors. Thus, individuals who have highly stressed and overloaded circuits may be phenotypically normal but have an increased risk for development of future anxiety disorders. This is known as a "presymptomatic" state.

Progression from Stress Sensitization

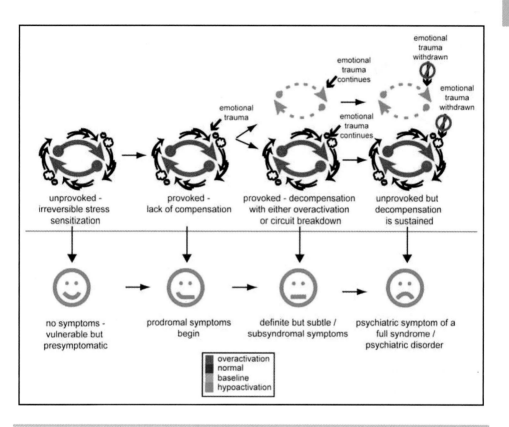

FIGURE 1.15. This figure shows the progression from stress sensitization to psychiatric symptoms. Stress sensitized circuits at rest are shown on the far left. In the absence of additional stressors, these overly activated circuits are clinically silent because they are able to compensate for the excessive activation. However, they are less efficient in their information processing than are normal, nonsensitized circuits. Under additional stress or emotional trauma, stress-sensitized circuits are hypothetically unable to compensate and begin to show signs of breakdown into subtle prodromal symptoms (middle left). With further emotional trauma, these failing circuits either do not compensate when they overly activate or even break down and fail to activate adequately, leading to the development of subsyndromal symptoms (middle right). Finally, with continuing emotional trauma, the malfunctioning circuits break down further; thereafter psychiatric symptoms not only develop but may persist even after withdrawal of the emotional trauma (far right).

Is All Stress Bad?

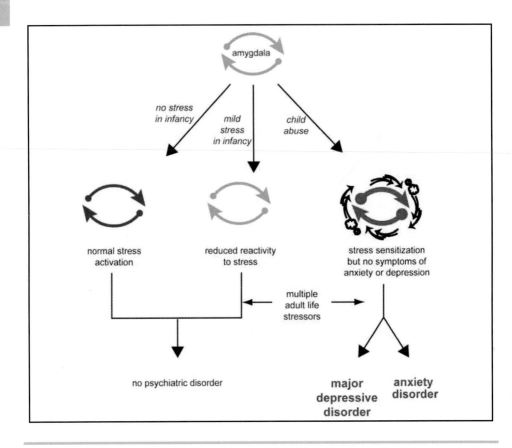

FIGURE 1.16. The experience of life stress can create stress sensitization and consequently increased risk for psychiatric illness, as shown in Figure 1.15. Interestingly, however, the degree of stress seems to make a difference, with only severe or overwhelming stress generally leading to sensitization (far right). In fact, exposure to mild stress in infancy may actually be protective: studies have shown that animals who have experienced mild stress in infancy may be less reactive to future stressors (middle) than animals not previously exposed to stress (left).

Stress Diathesis Model:
A Tale of Two Influences, Part 1

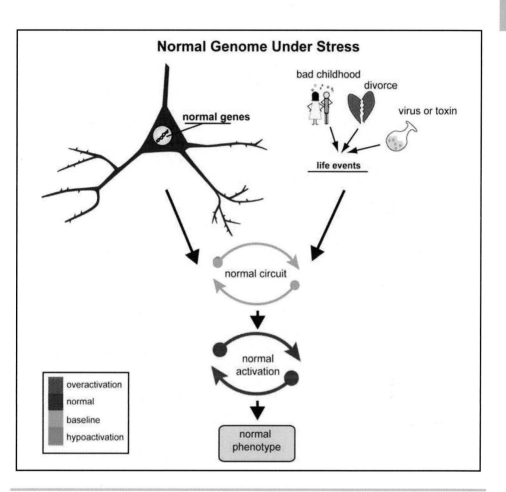

FIGURE 1.17. Exposure to stress isn't the whole story, however. Psychiatric symptoms often develop due both to genetic and environmental influences. This is known as the stress diathesis hypothesis.

Thus, although environmental stressors—such as childhood abuse, divorce, viruses, or toxins—can increase the risk, or diathesis, of developing a mental illness, individuals with a normal genome and thus normal circuits may experience only normal activation of circuits in response to these stressful events. Such individuals would not express a mental illness, exhibiting instead a normal phenotype with no adverse behavioral symptoms.

Stress Diathesis Model:
A Tale of Two Influences, Part 2

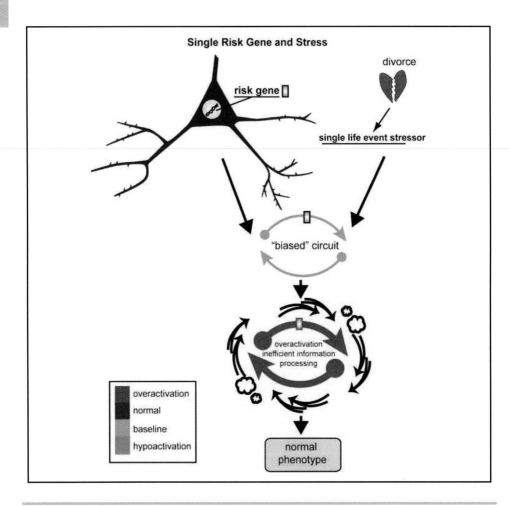

FIGURE 1.18. However, individuals with a risk gene for mental illness may experience inefficient information processing in the "biased" circuit in response to stress, increasing the likelihood of stress sensitization. This does not necessarily mean that behavioral symptoms will ensue. Genetically inefficient information processing may be behaviorally "silent" if it is compensated by overactivation via backup systems. In this case, the individual may still have a normal behavioral phenotype despite having an abnormal biological endophenotype. Thus, abnormal circuit activation may be detectable with functional brain scanning, but clinical interview would reveal no psychiatric symptoms.

Stahl's Illustrated

Stress Diathesis Model:
A Tale of Two Influences, Part 3

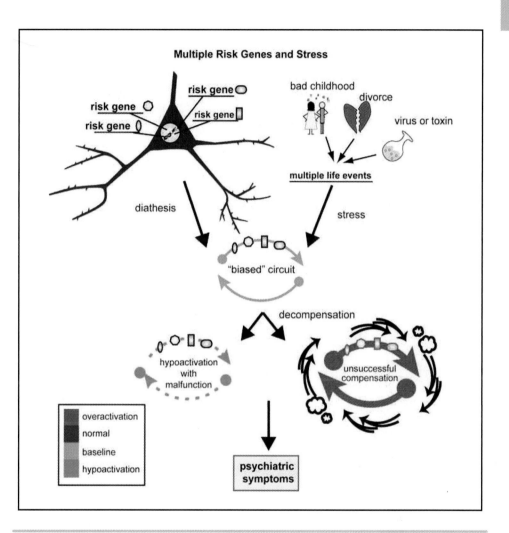

FIGURE 1.19. An individual with multiple stressors and multiple genetic risks may not have sufficient backup mechanisms to compensate for inefficient information processing within a genetically "biased" circuit. The circuit may either be unsuccessfully compensated by overactivation or it may break down and not activate at all. In either case, psychiatric symptoms would be likely to develop.

An Allegorical View of Stress Diathesis

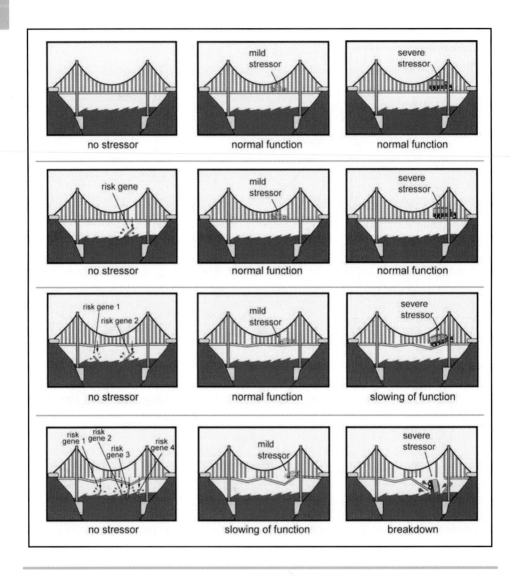

FIGURE 1.20. This representation summarizes the concept of stress diathesis, which was explained in Figures 1.17 through 1.19. Each suspension cable is analogous to a gene, while the vehicles that pass over the bridge represent types of environmental stressors.

Posttraumatic Stress Disorder (PTSD)

A surprisingly high percentage of the population will experience at least one traumatic event in their lifetime (trauma being defined as a frightening situation in which one experiences or witnesses the threat of death or injury). Although not all individuals exposed to traumatic events will develop psychopathology—in fact, most do not—a significant minority will, with potentially devastating consequences for them and their loved ones.

Posttraumatic stress disorder (PTSD) has a prevalence rate of 7–8%, with even higher rates for specific subpopulations (e.g., military personnel). It is a disorder with significant impact on functioning and quality of life and should be diagnosed and treated according to the best available evidence.

This chapter covers the clinical presentation of PTSD, including comorbidities and suicidality as well as its underlying risk factors and neurobiology.

PTSD:
An Historical Perspective

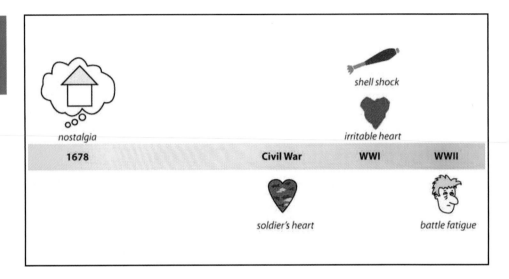

FIGURE 2.1. The psychological consequences of extremely stressful and dangerous situations such as warfare have been documented since ancient Roman times. It was not until the last thirty years, however, that those consequences were recognized as anything more than weakness of character in the individuals who suffered from them. Though PTSD is not confined to war-related traumas, most evolutions of its name and hypothesized etiology have derived from examination of military experiences.

The first modern conceptualization of posttraumatic stress symptoms was described in 1678 as nostalgia and attributed to homesickness on the part of soldiers. Nearly two hundred years later, advances in modern weaponry contributed to such a large proportion of American Civil War soldiers exhibiting stress-related ailments—soldier's heart—that the first military hospital for the insane was established. Further advances in weapon technology in the First World War led to the proposed etiology of brain concussion caused by exploding shells, and hence the term shell shock. Other conceptualizations of posttraumatic symptoms at that time included irritable heart (overstimulation of the sympathetic nervous system) and war neurosis (Freud's suggestion that soldiers were reconciling their traumatic experiences in their minds). By the end of World War I posttraumatic stress was no longer attributed to physical brain injury, and by World War II the term battle fatigue had emerged, again with the implication that it represented weakness.

PTSD:

An Historical Perspective (cont.)

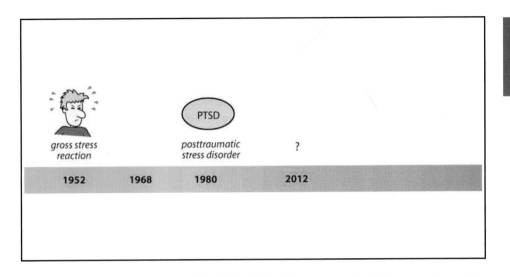

FIGURE 2.1 (CONT.). The first edition of the DSM contained the entry "gross stress reaction" under the category "transient situational personality disturbances." This was not considered a true diagnosis but rather a temporary state experienced by a "normal" person who had experienced great or unusual stress. This entry was eliminated from DSM-II, with no corresponding replacement. Advances in the field of psychiatry, coinciding with the return of hundreds of thousands of Vietnam War veterans suffering from posttraumatic stress, ultimately led to the inclusion of PTSD in the third edition of the DSM, published in 1980. Since then the diagnosis has been retained, although revisions to criteria have occurred, most notably with respect to the definition of a traumatic event. Further revisions are likely, as planning for DSM-V is heavily underway and debate in the literature abounds regarding how PTSD should be defined, described, and classified.

Criteria Controversies and the Future of PTSD

Current Criteria	Considerations
A. Exposure to traumatic event	Is this necessary?
1) Experience, witness, or be confronted with actual or threatened death or serious injury or threat to physical integrity of self or others	Too restrictive? Not restrictive enough? Is indirect exposure sufficient?
2) Intense fear, helplessness, horror	Does this add to the diagnosis?
B. Persistent reexperiencing of the event (1 of 5 possible manifestations)	Does this add to the diagnosis? (does not distinguish between PTSD and normative response to trauma)
C. Avoidance of stimuli associated with the trauma / numbing of general responsiveness (3 of 7 symptoms)	Strong predictor of PTSD Too stringent and restrictive?
D. Persistent hyperarousal (2 of 5 symptoms)	Does this add to the diagnosis? (does not distinguish between PTSD and normative response to trauma, not specific to PTSD)

FIGURE 2.2. The current diagnostic criteria for PTSD (DSM-IV-TR) are shown here. A diagnosis of PTSD depends on exposure to a traumatic event (A) and development of symptoms related to that event (B through D). There is some degree of controversy surrounding each of these criteria groups; however, most controversy is with respect to criterion A. Debate exists surrounding the type of qualifying traumatic event, the degree of exposure required, and even whether a traumatic event should be required at all. Accordingly, the DSM-V posttraumatic and dissociative disorders sub-work group is considering (1) whether/how to revise A1; (2) whether to retain or revise A2; (3) whether to revise, reduce, or expand B, C, and D; (4) whether PTSD should be reclassified with adjustment and dissociative disorders rather than with anxiety disorders; (5) whether to add any new proposed trauma-related disorders; and (6) how to create developmentally sensitive criteria.

Clinical Picture of PTSD

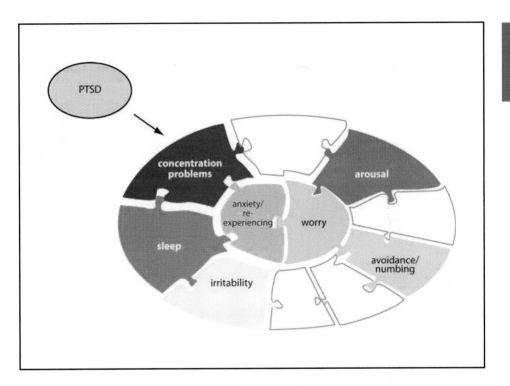

FIGURE 2.3. Characteristic symptoms of PTSD are shown here. Of 17 total diagnostic symptoms, only 6 are required for a diagnosis; thus it is possible that two individuals with PTSD could express quite divergent symptom profiles. Nonetheless, the majority of patients with PTSD will exhibit anxiety related to reexperiencing of the traumatic event (intrusive thoughts, dreams, flashbacks), hyperarousal and startle responses (as well as corresponding worry about experiencing such responses), avoidance behaviors, feelings of alienation, emotional numbing, anger and irritability, and sleep difficulties including nightmares.

Common Comorbidities

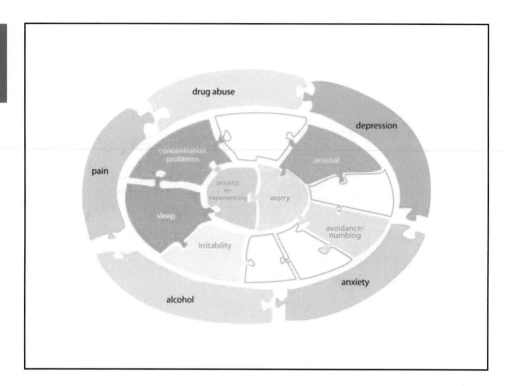

FIGURE 2.4. It is more common than not for a patient with PTSD to have at least one comorbid psychiatric disorder, with the most frequent comorbidities being major depressive disorder, alcohol dependence, drug abuse, and other anxiety disorders. Chronic pain can also be a frequent comorbidity, particularly following traumatic events involving injury (see Figure 2.10).

It is common for patients with PTSD to have a psychiatric history prior to exposure to a traumatic event; however, it is also common for a comorbid disorder to be diagnosed subsequent to onset of PTSD. Some argue that the rates of comorbidity in PTSD are artificially high owing to the degree of symptom overlap between PTSD and depression/other anxiety disorders. This is an important consideration warranting further investigation, though from a clinical practice perspective it may be most important to recognize the symptoms that patients experience, regardless of the disorder to which they might be attributed.

Suicide Risk

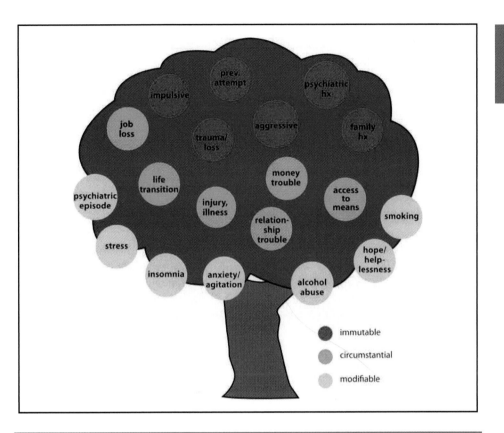

FIGURE 2.5. Rates of suicide ideation, attempts, and completions are alarmingly high in PTSD, regardless of the type of trauma experienced. PTSD is the only anxiety disorder that independently predicts suicidal behavior, though risk may also be increased in patients with comorbid disorders, particularly depression. The high rate of suicidal behavior in PTSD may not be surprising considering the overlap between recognized risk factors for suicidality, shown here, and the symptoms and associated features of PTSD. In particular, research shows that disorders characterized by extreme anxiety and agitation—such as PTSD—as well as those characterized by poor impulse control—such as substance use disorders, commonly comorbid with PTSD—are the strongest predictors of suicide attempts among psychiatric disorders. Although many risk factors for suicidality are difficult or impossible to address (depicted as "high-hanging" fruit), certain factors, many of which are relevant to PTSD, can be addressed ("low-hanging" fruit).

Risk Factors that Predict PTSD

STRONG	MODERATE	???
Psychiatric history	Life stress	Trauma type
Childhood abuse	Lack of social support	Small hippocampus
Family psychiatric history	Other previous trauma	Hypocortisolism
	Other adverse childhood experience	Genetic polymorphisms
	Trauma severity	

TABLE 2.1. PTSD's dependence on a causal event creates the complication of two potential sets of risk factors: those for exposure to a traumatic event and those for development of PTSD following exposure to a traumatic event. The risk factors shown here have been documented to predict PTSD, but some (e.g., psychiatric history) may also be risk factors for trauma exposure.

Early Life Stress as a Risk Factor for PTSD

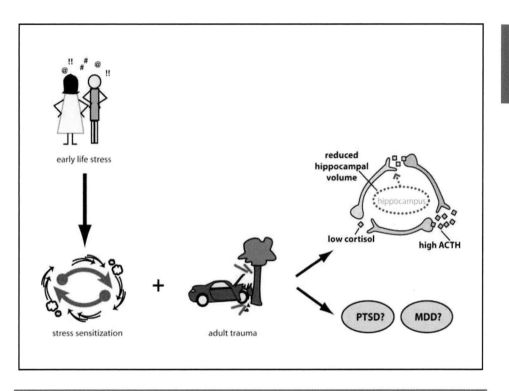

FIGURE 2.6. Stressful experiences in early life, such as childhood abuse or neglect, can have long-term negative consequences (see Figures 1.13 through 1.20). At a neurophysiological level, exposure to early life stress can lead to dysregulation of the HPA axis that may be characterized by either hypo- or hyperactive stress responses (see Figure 1.6). Specifically, individuals with a history of early life stress demonstrate exaggerated ACTH release and reduced cortisol release in response to stressors. Hippocampal atrophy has also been documented in this population, as has reduced levels of brain-derived neurotrophic factor (BDNF).

At a phenotypic level, these neurophysiological alterations are associated with increased risk for development of mental illnesses, most notably major depressive disorder (MDD) and PTSD.

PTSD and the HPA Axis

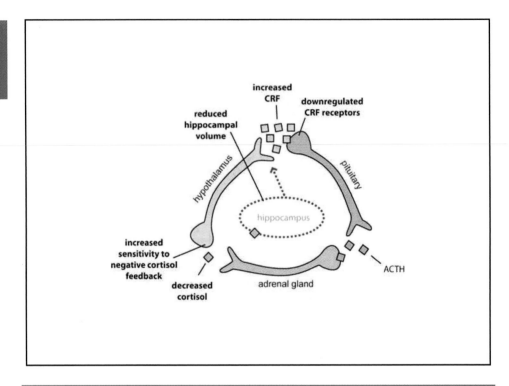

FIGURE 2.7. In PTSD, several abnormalities in HPA axis function have been identified, including increased CRF, downregulation of CRF receptors, decreased cortisol levels, and increased sensitivity to negative cortisol feedback. In addition, reduced hippocampal volume has been documented.

Reduced Hippocampal Volume and Stress:
Cause or Effect?

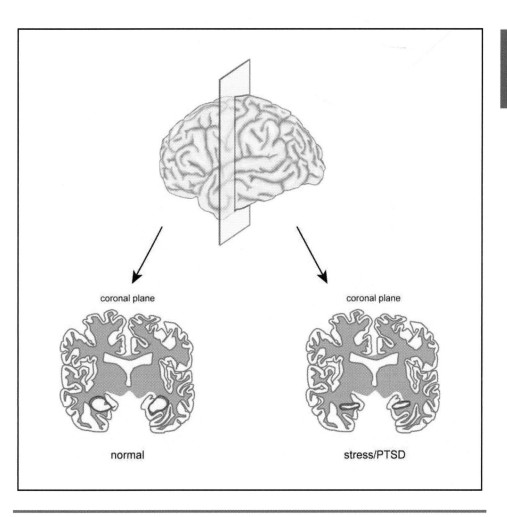

FIGURE 2.8. It is unknown whether reduced hippocampal volume may be a marker of preexisting vulnerability to stress, a structural consequence of stress, or both. Reduced hippocampal volume has been found in adult maltreatment-related PTSD, but not in childhood maltreatment-related PTSD, suggesting that it is a consequence of stress that occurs over time. On the other hand, a twin study in combat-related PTSD suggests that smaller hippocampal volume may be a risk factor for PTSD development.

Genetic Risk Factors

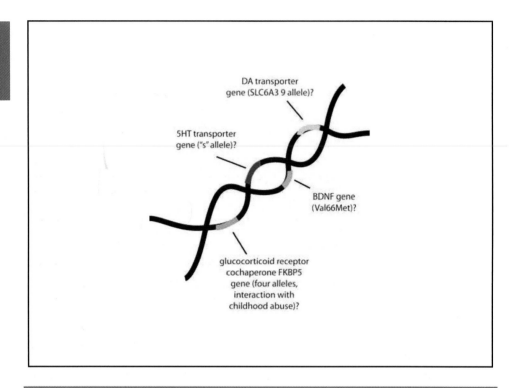

FIGURE 2.9. Isolating specific genetic influences in PTSD can be difficult, as it, like other mental illnesses, is a complex disorder characterized by multiple genetic and environmental risk factors (Table 2.1). Several polymorphisms that may increase risk for PTSD are under investigation. These include the SLC6A3 9 repeat allele in the dopamine transporter gene, the "s" allele in the serotonin transporter gene (see Figures 3.3 and 3.4), Val66Met in the BDNF gene, and multiple polymorphisms in the FKBP5 gene. FKBP5 is a glucocorticoid receptor cochaperone; thus polymorphisms in its gene could affect HPA axis functionality, which is altered in both child abuse survivors and individuals with PTSD (Figures 2.6 and 2.7). In fact, four single nucleotide polymorphisms in the FKBP5 gene seem to interact with severity of child abuse to predict adult PTSD symptoms. Further investigation into this and other potential candidate genes is ongoing.

Neuroimaging Findings in PTSD

Brain Region	Functional	Structural	Potential Implications
Amygdala	↑		Exaggerated fear response
rACC	↓	↓ volume	Deficits in extinction, emotion regulation, attention, contextual processing
dACC	↑		Exaggerated fear learning
Hippocampus	↑↓	↓ volume	Deficits in contextual processing Intrusive memories
Insular cortex	↑↓	↓ volume	Increased anxiety proneness

rACC: rostral anterior cingulate cortex. dACC: dorsal anterior cingulate cortex.

TABLE 2.2. There is no existing biomarker for assessing risk for, diagnosing, or charting progression of PTSD. We can still be informed, however, by neuroimaging and other studies that have shown neurobiological abnormalities in patients with PTSD. Summarized here is the current neurobiological evidence, including potential clinical implications of those findings (those with the strongest evidence are shown in green). As with reduced hippocampal volume (included here and discussed in Figure 2.8), it remains unknown whether these neurobiological changes in PTSD patients reflect risk factors for or consequences of the disorder.

Relationship Between Trauma Type and PTSD

TABLE 2.3.

Men			Women		
Trauma	Lifetime Prevalence	Probability of PTSD	Trauma	Lifetime Prevalence	Probability of PTSD
Witness	↑	↓	Natural disaster	↑	↓
Accident	↑	↓	Witness	↑	↓
Threat with weapon	↑	↓	Accident	↑	↓
Natural disaster	↑	↓	Molestation	↑	↑
Combat	↓	↑	Rape	↔	↑
Childhood physical abuse	↓	↑	Physical Attack	↓	↑
Molestation	↓	↑	Threat with weapon	↓	↑
Childhood neglect	↓	↑	Childhood physical abuse	↓	↑
Rape	↓	↑	Childhood neglect	↓	↑

Traumatic events are listed by lifetime prevalence, descending order. Individuals may have experienced more than one trauma; probability of a trauma type's association with PTSD was assessed for the primary (most upsetting) trauma. Traumas indicated as having relatively high lifetime prevalence or probability of PTSD (up arrow in red) have rates of 12% or higher. Those indicated as having relatively low lifetime prevalence or probability of PTSD (down arrow in green) have rates of 7% or lower. Trauma types with the highest probability of PTSD for each gender are written in red.

Relationship Between Trauma Type and PTSD (cont.)

TABLE 2.3. The majority of people have experienced a traumatic event (as defined in DSM). In addition, individuals who have experienced a traumatic event are actually likely to have experienced more than one. The most frequently experienced traumas are witnessing the death or extreme injury of another person, being involved in a natural disaster such as fire or flood, and being involved in a life-threatening accident. Although these are the most frequent trauma types across genders, men are more likely to experience them; men are also more likely than women to be threatened with a weapon, be physically attacked, or engage in combat, and in fact are more likely to experience a trauma overall. Women are more likely than men to be molested, raped, or physically abused or neglected as a child.

The majority of individuals exposed to a trauma do not develop PTSD. In addition, the most commonly experienced traumatic events are not the ones most associated with PTSD. In fact, although rape is the trauma type with the lowest lifetime prevalence in men it is associated with the highest probability of PTSD. Combat, childhood neglect, and childhood physical abuse are also associated with high probability of PTSD in men. In women, the trauma types associated with the highest probability of PTSD are childhood physical abuse, rape, being threatened with a weapon, and molestation.

Although men are more likely than women to experience a traumatic event, women are more likely to experience a trauma associated with a high probability of developing PTSD. Women may also be more likely than men to meet criteria for PTSD following a traumatic event. Both of these factors may contribute to the higher rate of PTSD in women than in men.

Although it is interesting to evaluate the relationship between trauma type and PTSD, it is not currently clear what influence trauma type has on the risk for exposure to future stressors, the risk for development of PTSD, or the symptom expression of PTSD.

PTSD and Chronic Pain

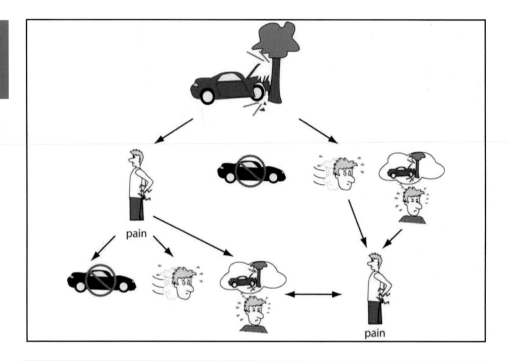

FIGURE 2.10. Many traumatic events that can lead to PTSD (e.g., accidents, combat, physical attack) can also result in physical injury, and in many cases the pain associated with such injury may become chronic. In fact, PTSD and chronic pain are common comorbidities following a traumatic event. The extent and nature of the relationship between PTSD and pain is not known, but there is some evidence that PTSD can drive pain and that pain can drive PTSD—in other words, that there is a mutual maintenance relationship between the two.

In theory, if pain occurred in conjunction with a traumatic event, then subsequent pain could trigger distressing memories of the event that in turn lead to arousal and avoidance. Arousal can cause muscle tension that may exacerbate pain; the pain itself may also be so distressing that it leads to avoidance. This model is supported by a recent longitudinal study in which reexperiencing and arousal symptoms at the time of a traumatic event predicted pain at three months; further, reexperiencing and arousal at three months predicted pain at twelve months. In turn, pain at baseline predicted arousal at three months, while pain at three months predicted reexperiencing, arousal, and avoidance at twelve months.

Neurotransmitter Systems as Pharmacological Targets for PTSD

In Chapter 1 we matched the core symptoms of anxiety disorders with the brain circuits that hypothetically mediate them, and illustrated how those circuits can become sensitized and increase risk for a psychiatric disorder such as PTSD. Chapter 3 reviews the major neurotransmitter systems that regulate functioning within those brain circuits, and that are therefore potential targets of pharmacologic action in the treatment of PTSD.

The Neurotransmitters of Fear and Worry

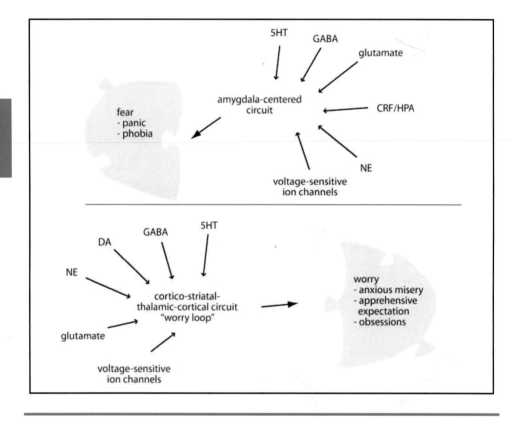

FIGURE 3.1. The major chemical players in amygdala-centered circuits include serotonin (5HT), gamma-aminobutyric acid (GABA), norepinephrine (NE), glutamate, corticotrophin releasing factor (CRF), and other hormones involved in HPA axis function. 5HT, GABA, NE, and glutamate are also central to functioning in the CSTC loops of worry, as is dopamine (DA). In addition, voltage-sensitive ion channels are involved in neurotransmission in all of these circuits. Each of these neurotransmitters systems are discussed in turn on the following pages.

Serotonergic Pathways

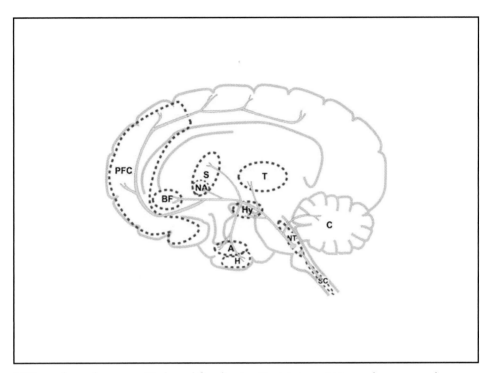

PFC: prefrontal cortex. BF: basal forebrain. S: striatum. NA: nucleus accumbens.
T: thalamus. Hy: hypothalamus. A: amygdala. H: hippocampus. NT: brain neurotransmitter center. SC: spinal cord. C: cerebellum.

FIGURE 3.2. These are the major serotonergic projections in the brain. As shown,
serotonergic neurons innervate the amygdala and the prefrontal cortex, two regions
essential to anxiety and worry. Serotonin has also been implicated in other symptoms associated with PTSD, including emotional numbing, irritability, and suicidality.
In fact, many of the pharmacologic agents used to treat PTSD have as their central
mechanism the modulation of serotonergic neurotransmission (see Chapters 4 and
5). There is some evidence for altered serotonin neurotransmission in PTSD, including
decreased serum concentrations and decreased density of platelet serotonin uptake
sites. Further evidence implicating serotonin in anxiety and fear comes from genetic
studies looking at the serotonin transporter (SERT) gene and amygdala reactivity.

SERT Genotype and Amygdala Activation, Part 1

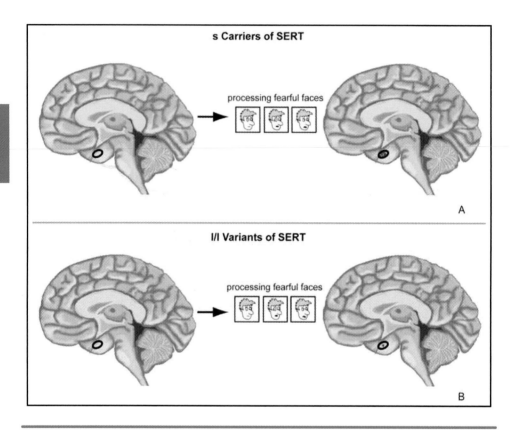

FIGURE 3.3. Genetic research has shown that the type of SERT (serotonin transporter) one has can affect how active the amygdala is in response to fearful stimuli. A polymorphism in the gene that codes for SERT yields two alleles, one long ("l") and one short ("s"). Carriers of the s allele make fewer copies of SERT, have lower amounts of SERT reuptake activity, and have higher amounts of synaptic serotonin. Functional neuroimaging data show that s carriers also have greater amygdala reactivity to fearful faces (A) than do those with the l/l variant (B).

SERT Genotype and Amygdala Activation, Part 2

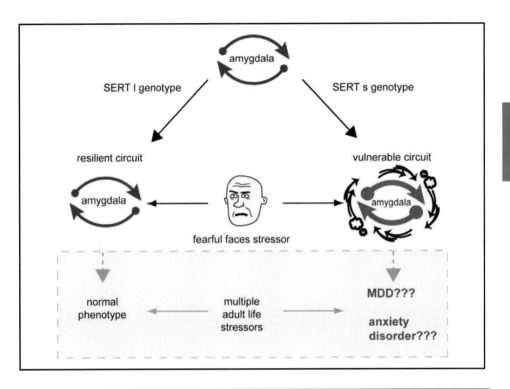

FIGURE 3.4. Another way of saying this may be that the l/l genotype leads to a "resilient" circuit that can process fearful or stressful stimuli efficiently, whereas the s genotype leads to a "vulnerable" circuit that overreacts in response to fearful or stressful stimuli. The relationship between SERT variants and amygdala reactivity has been demonstrated in multiple studies as well as a recent meta-analysis, and is further supported by results of a recent fear-conditioning study in which only s carriers developed conditioned startle potentiation.

The clinical implications of the SERT variant/amygdala reactivity relationship are not yet known, however. A recent meta-analysis of SERT studies found no association between SERT variant and risk for depression, neither as a main effect nor as an interaction effect between genotype and stressful life events. Thus, although it has been posited that overactivation of circuits in s carriers may confer greater risk of developing a mood or anxiety disorder in the context of multiple life stressors, current evidence does not support this.

Potential Targets for Modulating Serotonergic Neurotransmission, Part 1

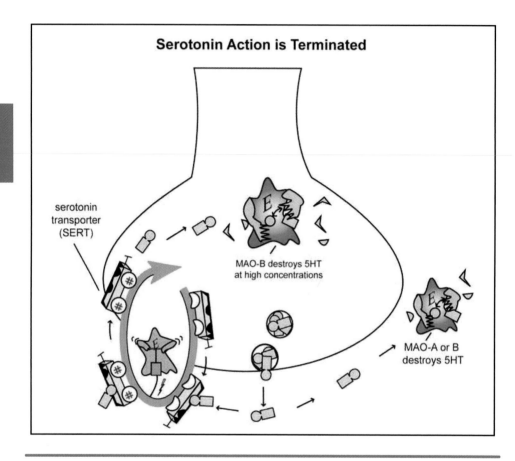

FIGURE 3.5. Given the clear link between the 5HT system and amygdala activity, it is not surprising that many of the pharmacologic agents used to treat anxiety are primarily serotonergic in mechanism. Shown here and in Figure 3.6 are some of the potential targets for modulating the serotonin system. Specific agents that act at these sites are discussed in Chapters 4 and 5.

Serotonin can have its synaptic action terminated by the serotonin transporter, SERT, which transports serotonin molecules back into the presynaptic neuron for reuse (see Chapter 4 for agents acting at SERT). Serotonin can also be destroyed by mono-amine oxidase (MAO) enzymes, which convert serotonin molecules into an inactive derivative (see Figure 5.7 for agents acting at MAO enzymes).

Potential Targets for Modulating Serotonergic Neurotransmission, Part 2

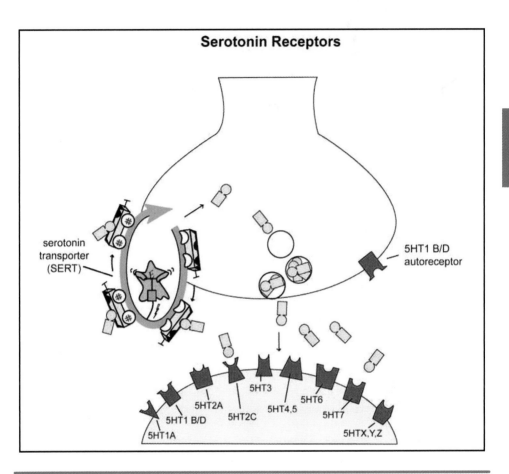

FIGURE 3.6. Pre- and postsynaptic serotonin receptors are shown here. On the presynaptic side, in addition to the 5HT transporter (see Figure 3.5), there is a key presynaptic 5HT receptor (5HT1B/D) that functions as an autoreceptor to regulate 5HT release. There are also several postsynaptic 5HT receptors (5HT1A, 5HT1B/D, 5HT2A, 5HT2C, 5HT3, 5HT4, 5HT6, 5HT7, and many others denoted by 5HTX,Y,Z) as shown here.

Noradrenergic Pathways

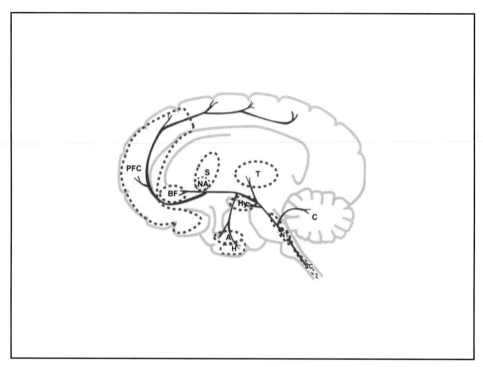

PFC: prefrontal cortex. BF: basal forebrain. S: striatum. NA: nucleus accumbens. T: thalamus. Hy: hypothalamus. A: amygdala. H: hippocampus. NT: brain neurotransmitter center. SC: spinal cord. C: cerebellum.

FIGURE 3.7. These are the major noradrenergic projections in the brain. Like serotonergic neurons, noradrenergic neurons innervate the amygdala and the prefrontal cortex, both of which are essential to anxiety and worry. In addition, noradrenergic neurons originate in the locus coeruleus, which is responsible for the autonomic output of fear (see Figure 1.4).

Potential Noradrenergic Mechanisms for Novel Anxiolytics

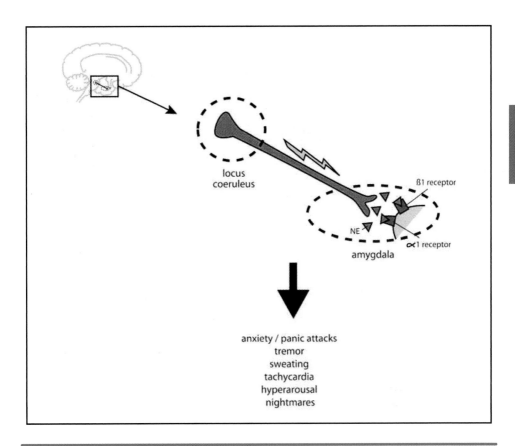

FIGURE 3.8. Noradrenergic hyperactivation can lead to anxiety, panic attacks, tremors, sweating, tachycardia, hyperarousal, and nightmares. Such autonomic reactivity at the time of exposure to a traumatic event may be associated with risk of developing PTSD. Alpha 1 and beta 1 adrenergic receptors may be specifically involved in these reactions (see Figures 3.10, 5.16, and 5.33).

Potential Targets for Modulating Noradrenergic Neurotransmission, Part 1

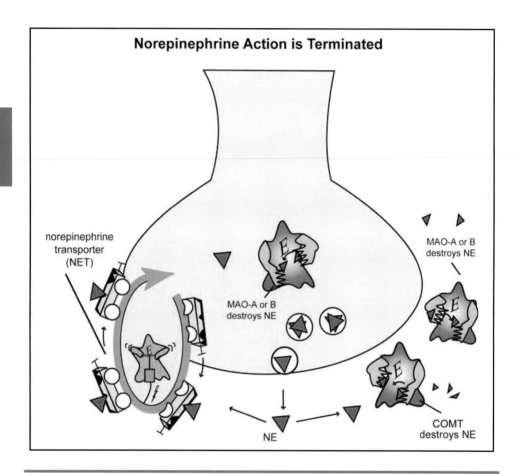

FIGURE 3.9. Shown here and in Figure 3.10 are some of the potential pharmaco-logic targets for modulating the noradrenergic system. Specific agents that act at these sites are discussed in Chapters 4 and 5.

Norepinephrine can have its synaptic action terminated by the norepinephrine transporter (NET), which transports norepinephrine molecules back into the presyn-aptic neuron for reuse (see Chapter 4 for agents acting at NET). Norepinephrine can also be destroyed by MAO enzymes, which convert norepinephrine molecules into an inactive derivative (see Figure 5.7 for agents acting at MAO enzymes).

Potential Targets for Modulating Noradrenergic Neurotransmission, Part 2

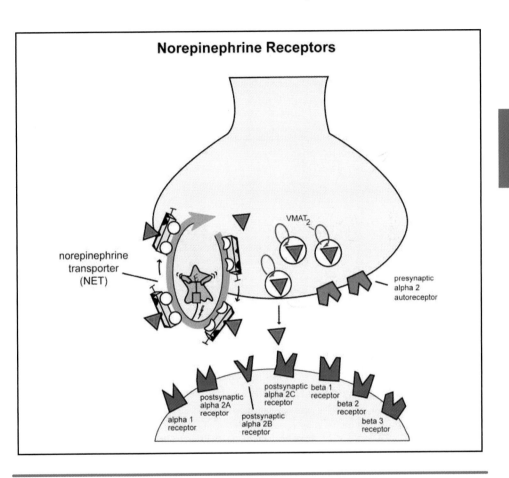

FIGURE 3.10. Pre- and postsynaptic norepinephrine receptors are shown here. On the presynaptic side, in addition to the NE transporter (see Figure 3.9), there is a key presynaptic NE receptor (alpha 2) that functions as an autoreceptor to regulate NE release. There are also several postsynaptic NE receptors (alpha 1, 2A, 2B, and 2C; beta 1, 2, and 3) as shown here. Alpha 1 and beta 1 receptors may be of particular importance to the treatment of anxiety (see Figures 5.16 and 5.33).

GABA "Pathways"

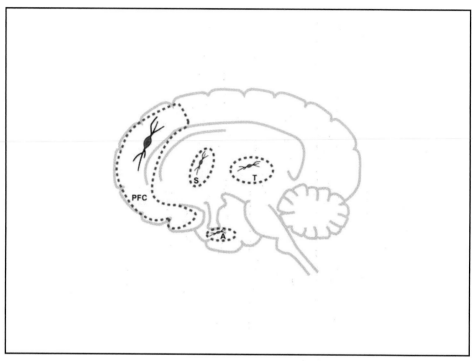

PFC: prefrontal cortex. S: striatum. T: thalamus. A: amygdala.

FIGURE 3.11. GABA is the major inhibitory neurotransmitter in the brain, regulating and reducing the activity of many neurons, including neurons in the amygdala and within CSTC loops. GABA therefore plays a key role in the experience and expression of anxiety, and can potentially be modulated in order to reduce anxiety. Shown on the following pages are some of the potential pharmacologic targets for modulating the GABA-ergic system. Specific agents that act at these sites are discussed in Figures 5.11 and 5.37.

Potential Targets for Modulating GABA-ergic Neurotransmission

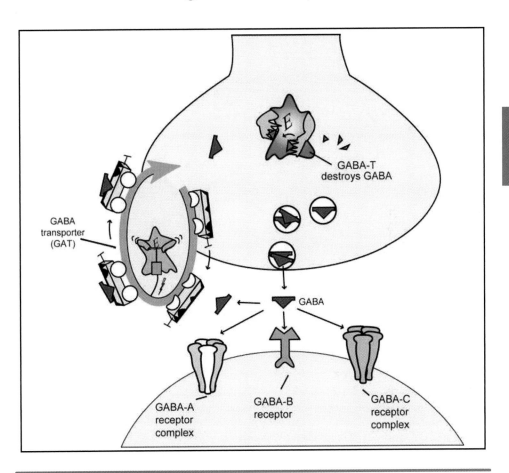

FIGURE 3.12. GABA can have its synaptic action terminated by the GABA transporter (GAT), which transports GABA molecules back into the presynaptic neuron for reuse, or by the enzyme GABA transaminase (GABA-T), which converts GABA in the presynaptic bouton into an inactive substance.

In addition to the GABA transporter, there are three major types of postsynaptic GABA receptors: GABA-A, GABA-B, and GABA-C. GABA-A and -C receptors are ligand-gated ion channels that form part of an inhibitory chloride channel, while GABA-B receptors are G protein-linked and can couple with calcium or potassium channels. GABA-A receptors are particularly relevant to anxiety and to the anxiolytic effects of benzodiazepines, and are discussed in more detail in Figure 5.10.

Glutamate Pathways

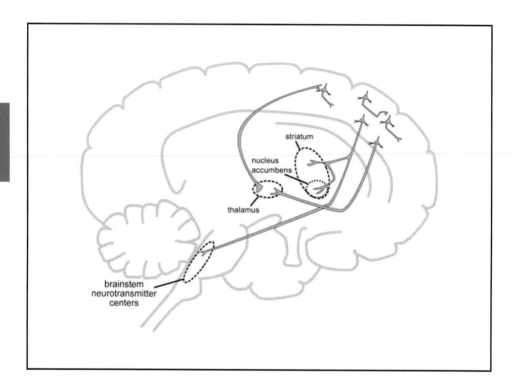

FIGURE 3.13. While GABA is the major inhibitory neurotransmitter in the brain (Figures 3.11 and 3.12), glutamate is the major excitatory neurotransmitter. Shown here are the main glutamatergic projections in the brain. Glutamate is a major player in communication between the prefrontal cortex (PFC) and other brain regions, and is particularly involved in CSTC loops.

Unlike GABA, which has had a recognized role in anxiety and its treatment for some time, glutamate has only recently received focus in this area. Shown on the following pages are some of the potential targets for modulating the glutamatergic system. Investigational agents that act at these sites are discussed in Figure 5.35.

Glutamate Receptors

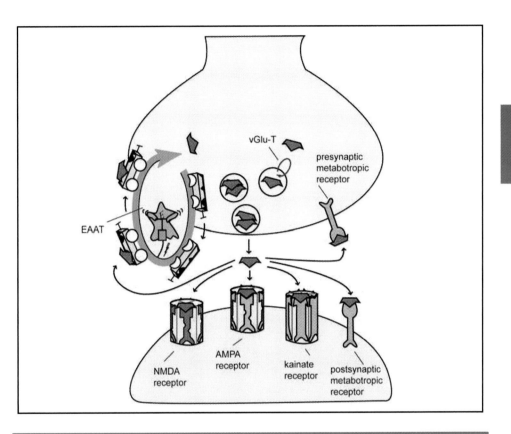

FIGURE 3.14. Pre- and postsynaptic glutamate receptors are shown here. The excitatory amino acid transporter (EAAT) clears excess glutamate from synapses and transports it back into the presynaptic neuron. Metabotropic glutamate receptors (mGluR) are linked to G-proteins and can occur either pre- or postsynaptically, with presynaptic mGluRs acting as autoreceptors to regulate glutamate release. Three other types of postsynaptic glutamate receptors are linked to ion channels and are named for the agonists that bind to them: NMDA (N-methyl-D-aspartate), AMPA (alpha-amino-3-hydroxy-5-methyl-4-isoxazolepropionic acid), and kainate. Glutamate's actions at NMDA receptors are dependent in part upon the presence of a cotransmitter, either glycine or d-serine, which are produced in nearby neurons (glycine) or glial cells (d-serine).

Voltage-Sensitive Ion Channels

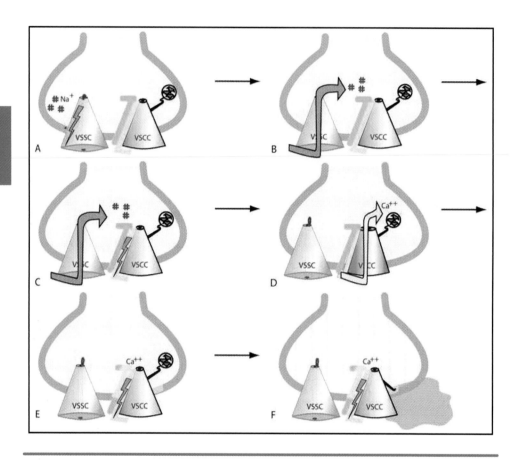

FIGURE 3.15. Excitatory neurotransmission may also be modulated by targeting voltage-sensitive ion channels, which are integrally involved in the process of neurotransmission, as shown here (see Figure 5.9 for agents acting at voltage-sensitive ion channels).

An action potential is sent to the axon terminal via voltage-sensitive sodium channels (VSSC) along the axon. The sodium released by those channels triggers a VSSC at the axon terminal to open (A), allowing sodium influx into the presynaptic neuron (B). This changes the electrical charge of the voltage-sensitive calcium channel (VSCC) (C), causing it to open and allow calcium influx (D). As the intraneuronal concentration of calcium increases (E), the synaptic vesicle is caused to dock and merge with the presynaptic membrane, leading to neurotransmitter release (F).

CRF and Other Stress Hormones

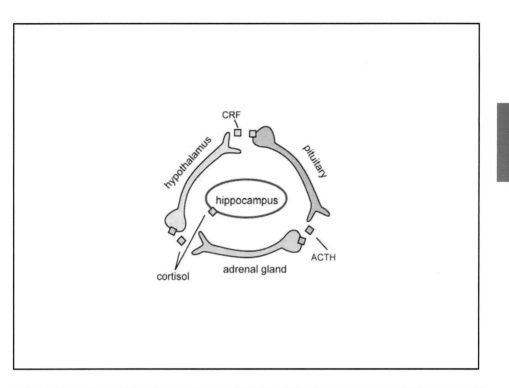

FIGURE 3.16. The central role of the HPA axis in stress responses (Figure 1.6) makes it logical that it would be involved in anxiety disorders, and this is in fact substantiated by evidence of HPA axis abnormalities in PTSD (Figure 2.7). Receptors and neurotransmitters within the HPA axis are therefore potential targets for pharmacological action in PTSD (investigational agents acting at these sites are discussed in Figures 5.34 and 5.36).

Dopamine and the PFC

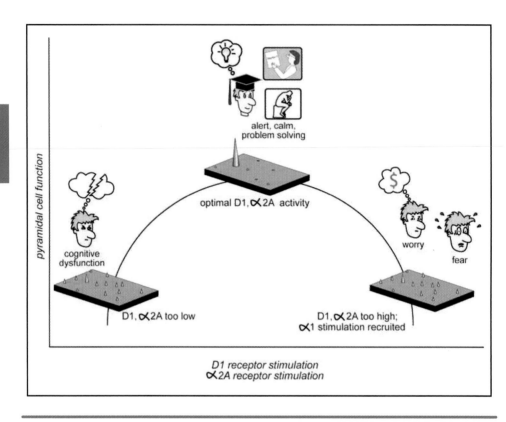

alert, calm,
problem solving

optimal D1, α2A activity

cognitive
dysfunction

worry

fear

D1, α2A too low

D1, α2A too high;
α1 stimulation recruited

pyramidal cell function

D1 receptor stimulation
α2A receptor stimulation

FIGURE 3.17. Dopamine is integral to functioning in the PFC, which is the brain region responsible (in conjunction with the thalamus and striatum) for worry symptoms such as apprehensive expectations, catastrophic thinking, and obsessions. Efficient functioning of the PFC requires a delicate balance of receptor stimulation, specifically alpha 2 receptors by NE and D1 receptors by DA.

In theory, NE increases incoming salient signals by allowing for increased connectivity of prefrontal networks, while DA decreases noise by preventing inappropriate connections from taking place. Cortical pyramidal cell function is optimal when stimulation of both alpha 2A and D1 receptors is moderate (top of curve). If stimulation at these receptors is too low (left), all incoming signals are the same, preventing a person from focusing on one single task. When stimulation is too high (right), the signals get scrambled as additional receptors are recruited, again misguiding a person's attention and potentially leading to inappropriate worry.

Born Worried? COMT Genotype and PFC Activation

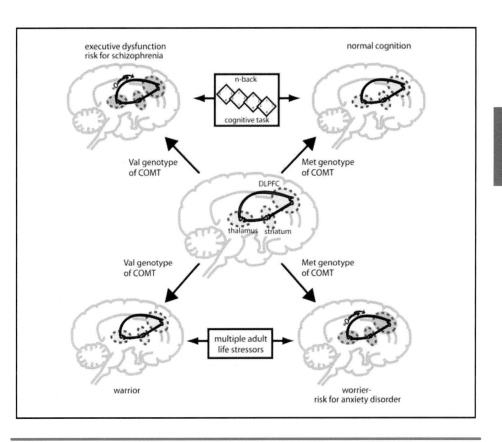

FIGURE 3.18. Dopamine levels in the PFC are regulated in large part by the enzyme catechol-O-methyl-transferase (COMT). A polymorphism in the gene that codes for COMT yields two alleles, "met" and "val," with the met/met genotype associated with lower COMT activity and thus higher DA levels. During cognitive tasks, this may be beneficial, allowing for normal activation (top right), whereas reduced DA with the val genotype may lead to inefficiency of cognitive information processing, potentially requiring more effort to perform less well (top left).

In the case of stress responses, however, the beneficial genotype may be reversed. That is, higher baseline DA levels with the met/met genotype combined with DA release in response to stress may cumulatively be excessive and contribute to worry and risk for anxiety disorders (bottom right). Those with the val genotype, on the other hand, may be less reactive to stress because COMT can destroy the excess dopamine (bottom left).

Conditioned Fear Extinction:
COMT

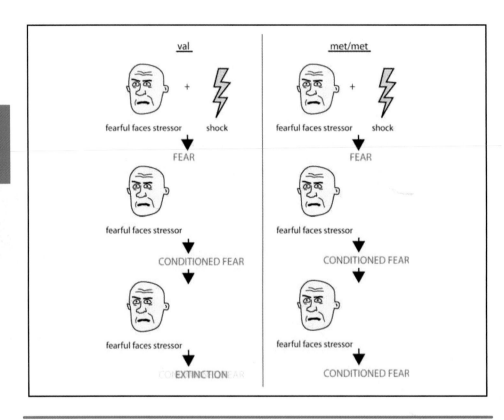

FIGURE 3.19. There is evidence not only that the variant of COMT may affect risk for anxiety disorders, but also that it may affect the likelihood that certain treatment will be effective. Specifically, a standard treatment for many anxiety disorders is exposure therapy, in which a feared stimulus is repeatedly presented without adverse consequences so that there is a progressive reduction of the response to the fear stimulus (discussed in more detail in Figure 6.2). This is known as fear extinction, and is a form of new learning (that the stimulus is not threatening) rather than elimination of the old conditioned fear.

In a preliminary study, individuals with the val genotype achieved extinction of a conditioned fear (measured by startle potentiation) to a fearful face that had originally been paired with shock (left). Those with the met/met genotype, on the other hand, did not achieve extinction, suggesting that too high levels of DA may have prevented efficient information processing in the PFC (right).

| Chapter 4

First-Line Medications for PTSD

First-line pharmacologic treatments for PTSD act predominantly on the serotonergic and, to a lesser extent, the noradrenergic systems. Specifically, these agents include the selective serotonin reuptake inhibitors (SSRIs) and the serotonin norepinephrine reuptake inhibitors (SNRIs). In this chapter, the mechanisms of action of agents within these two pharmacologic classes are explained, and a brief overview of clinical characteristics of each agent is provided in turn.

Symbols Used in this Chapter			
☠	Life-threatening or Dangerous Side Effects	👶	Pregnancy
⚠	Contraindications	♥	Cardiac Impairment
○	Tips and Pearls	🫘	Renal Impairment
👫	Children and Adolescents	🫀	Hepatic Impairment

Pharmacological Treatments

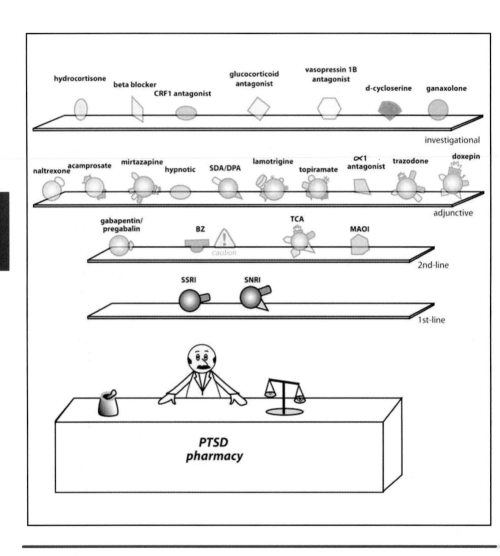

FIGURE 4.1. First-line medications for PTSD include the selective serotonin reuptake inhibitors (SSRIs) and serotonin norepinephrine reuptake inhibitors (SNRIs), with only paroxetine and sertraline approved by the Food and Drug Administration (FDA) for this indication. This figure will be used throughout the book to indicate where the various pharmacotherapies under discussion fall in the sequence of selecting treatments for PTSD.

Selective Serotonin Reuptake Inhibitors (SSRIs):
Mechanism of Action, Part 1

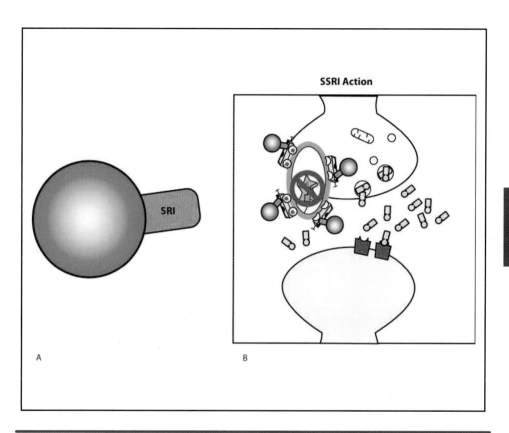

FIGURE 4.2. There are six agents within the SSRI class, all of which share the central feature of serotonin reuptake inhibition (SRI, indicated above in part A). These agents bind to the serotonin transporter (SERT), preventing serotonin (5HT) from being taken back up into the presynaptic neuron (B). However, the onset of action of SSRIs is delayed, suggesting that the therapeutic effects are actually related to downstream adaptive changes rather than acute actions at SERT.

Selective Serotonin Reuptake Inhibitors (SSRIs):
Mechanism of Action, Part 2

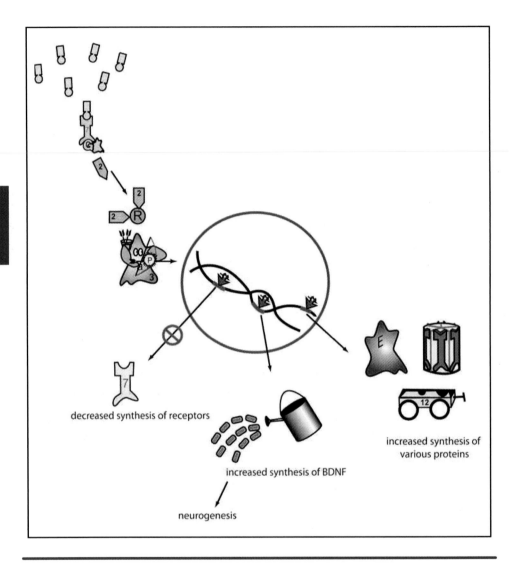

decreased synthesis of receptors

increased synthesis of various proteins

increased synthesis of BDNF

neurogenesis

FIGURE 4.3. The mechanism by which SSRIs may alleviate symptoms of PTSD is not truly understood. There is evidence that the increase in synaptic serotonin caused by SSRIs leads to a cascade of events that changes the expression of critical genes. This can affect synthesis of pre- and postsynaptic serotonin receptors as well as of other critical proteins. Thus the ultimate effects of SSRIs may be widespread.

Selective Serotonin Reuptake Inhibitors (SSRIs):
Mechanism of Action, Part 3

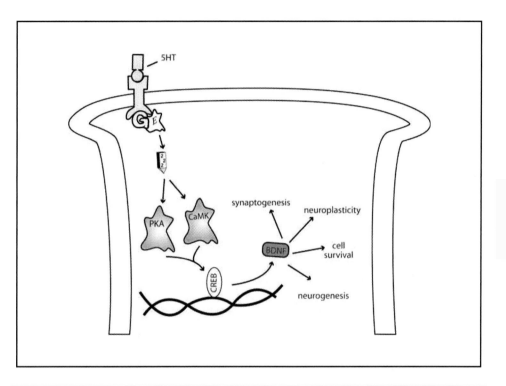

FIGURE 4.4. One particular effect of interest is that SSRIs can increase brain-derived neurotrophic factor (BDNF) levels, which are reduced in individuals exposed to extreme stress (see Figure 2.6) and may be related to hippocampal atrophy seen in PTSD (see Figure 2.8). Serotonin can increase the availability of BDNF by initiating signal transduction cascades that lead to its release. These actions may be further enhanced by therapeutic agents that boost serotonin (e.g., SSRIs).

Secondary Pharmacological Properties of SSRIs

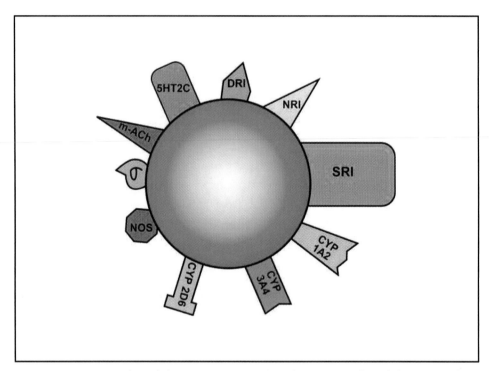

SRI: serotonin reuptake inhibition. NRI: norepinephrine reuptake inhibition. DRI: dopamine reuptake inhibition. 5HT2C: serotonin 2C antagonism. m-ACh: muscarinic/cholinergic antagonism. σ: sigma 1 receptor actions. NOS: nitric oxide synthetase inhibition. CYP 2D6: cytochrome p450 2D6 inhibition. CYP 3A4: cytochrome p450 3A4 inhibition. CYP 1A2: cytochrome p450 1A2 inhibition.

FIGURE 4.5. In addition to the shared feature of serotonin reuptake inhibition, each SSRI has different secondary properties that may contribute to their therapeutic and side effect profiles. The unique pharmacological and clinical properties of each of the six SSRIs (Table 4.1) are shown in Figures 4.6 through 4.17.

SSRIs

TABLE 4.1	
Agent	**Approved in PTSD**
paroxetine (Paxil, Aropax, Seroxat)	Yes
sertraline (Zoloft)	Yes
fluoxetine (Prozac, Serafem)	No
fluvoxamine (Luvox, Faverin)	No
citalopram (Celexa, Cipramil)	No
escitalopram (Lexapro, Cipralex)	No

Paroxetine

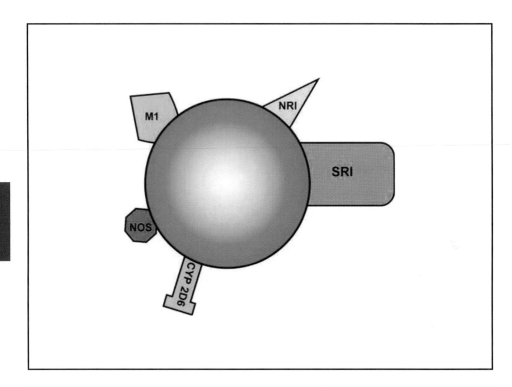

FIGURE 4.6. Paroxetine is used widely to treat anxiety disorders, and in fact is approved to treat all five major anxiety disorders, including PTSD. Paroxetine has anticholinergic effects (M1 muscarinic antagonism), which may contribute to its anxiolytic efficacy. In addition to this and SRI (serotonin reuptake inhibition) properties, paroxetine is a weak norepinephrine reuptake inhibitor (NRI), a nitric oxide synthetase (NOS) inhibitor, and a potent CYP450 2D6 inhibitor. Paroxetine is a substrate as well as an inhibitor of 2D6, which can lead to a rapid decline in plasma drug levels, contributing to the withdrawal symptoms experienced upon sudden discontinuation.

Paroxetine: Tips and Pearls

Dosing and Use

Formulations:
IR tablets: 10 mg scored, 20 mg scored, 30 mg, and 40 mg; CR tablets: 12.5 mg, 25 mg; liquid: 10mg/5 mL

Dosage Range:
IR 20–50 mg/day; CR 25–62.5 mg/day

Approved For:
Posttraumatic stress disorder, generalized anxiety disorder, panic disorder, social anxiety disorder, obsessive compulsive disorder, major depressive disorder, premenstrual dysphoric disorder

Side Effects and Safety

Weight Gain

unusual   not unusual   common   problematic

Sedation

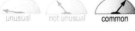
unusual   not unusual   common   problematic

 Rare: seizures, induction of mania, induction of suicidality in children, adolescents, and young adults

 Do not use with MAOIs, thioridazine, pimozide

Pearls

 Often preferred treatment of anxious depression and comorbid major depression and anxiety disorders; withdrawal effects may be more likely than with other SSRIs when discontinued; mild anticholinergic actions can enhance rapid onset of anxiolytic efficacy but also cause mild anticholinergic side effects

Special Populations

 Use with caution in children; watch for induction of mania or suicidal ideation

 Pregnancy risk category D (positive evidence of risk to human fetus; potential benefits may still justify its use during pregnancy)

 Preliminary research suggests that it is safe for patients with cardiac impairment

 Lower dose for renal impairment; maximum 40 mg/day (50 mg/day CR)

 Lower dose for hepatic impairment; maximum 40 mg/day (50 mg/day CR)

FIGURE 4.7. Dosing and safety information for paroxetine.

Sertraline

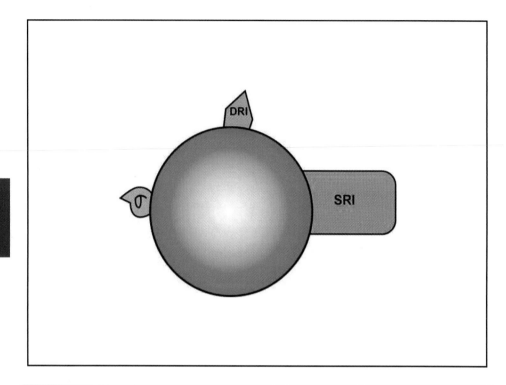

FIGURE 4.8. Sertraline is approved to treat multiple anxiety disorders, including PTSD. It has weak dopamine reuptake inhibition (DRI) properties and also binds to sigma 1 receptors, in addition to its SRI properties. While sigma 1 actions are not well understood, they may contribute to anxiolytic effects and may also be useful in psychotic depression. The actions at DAT may be weak, but perhaps only a small amount of DAT inhibition is enough to contribute to improvement of certain symptoms (e.g., concentration difficulties related to dopamine in the prefrontal cortex).

Sertraline: Tips and Pearls

Dosing and Use

Formulations:
Tablets: 25 mg, 50 mg scored, 100 mg; liquid: 20 mg/mL

Dosage Range:
50–200 mg/day

Approved For:
Posttraumatic stress disorder, panic disorder, social anxiety disorder, obsessive compulsive disorder, major depressive disorder, premenstrual dysphoric disorder

Side Effects and Safety

Weight Gain

unusual / not unusual / common / problematic

Sedation

unusual / not unusual / common / problematic

Rare: seizures, induction of mania, induction of suicidality in children, adolescents, and young adults

Do not use with MAOIs, thioridazine, pimozide; do not use liquid with disulfiram

Pearls

Often preferred for patients with low energy and hypersomnia; effective for comorbid depression; may initially cause increased anxiety or insomnia; sigma 1 actions may enhance anxiolytic effects

Special Populations

Use with caution in children; watch for activation of mania or suicidal ideation; approved for use in OCD

Pregnancy risk category C (some animal studies show adverse effects, no controlled studies in humans)

Proven cardiovascular safety in depressed patients with myocardial infarction or angina

No dose adjustment for renal impairment; not removed by hemo-dialysis

Lower dose by half or give less frequently for hepatic impairment

FIGURE 4.9. Dosing and safety information for sertraline.

Fluoxetine

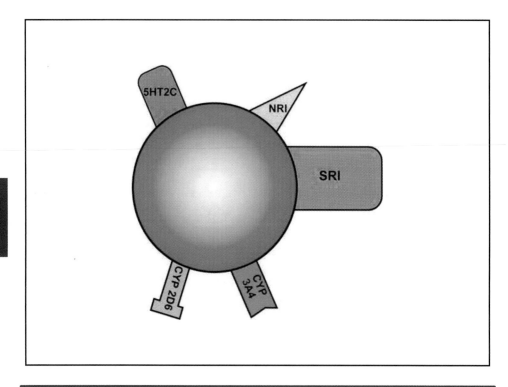

FIGURE 4.10. Fluoxetine is approved to treat multiple anxiety disorders, and though not approved has evidence of efficacy in PTSD. It has effects not only on the serotonin system via serotonin reuptake inhibition (SRI) but also on the norepinephrine and dopamine systems via weak norepinephrine reuptake inhibition (NRI) and antagonism at 5HT2C receptors. In brief, stimulation of 5HT2C receptors inhibits norepinephrine and dopamine release; thus antagonism of these receptors can lead to norepinephrine and dopamine release. This may contribute to increased anxiety and insomnia that is often experienced at initiation of treatment. Fluoxetine also inhibits CYP450 2D6 and 3A4. Fluoxetine has a long half-life, while its active metabolite has an even longer half-life; these factors may reduce the incidence of withdrawal symptoms following sudden discontinuation.

Fluoxetine: Tips and Pearls

Dosing and Use

Formulations:
Capsules: 10 mg, 20 mg, 40 mg; tablet: 10 mg; liquid: 20 mg/5 mL; weekly capsule: 90 mg

Dosage Range:
20–80 mg/day for anxiety

Approved For:
Panic disorder, obsessive compulsive disorder, major depressive disorder, premenstrual dysphoric disorder, bulimia nervosa, bipolar depression (in combination with olanzapine), treatment-resistant depression (in combination with olanzapine)

Side Effects and Safety

Weight Gain

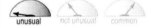
unusual   not unusual   common   problematic

Sedation

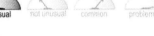
unusual   not unusual   common   problematic

 Rare: seizures, induction of mania, induction of suicidality in children, adolescents, and young adults

 Do not use with MAOIs, thioridazine, pimozide

Pearls

 Often preferred for patients with low energy and hypersomnia; effective for comorbid depression; may initially cause increased anxiety or insomnia, perhaps due to 5HT2C antagonism; not as well tolerated as other SSRIs as a monotherapy in anxiety disorders

Special Populations

 Use with caution in children; watch for activation of mania or suicidal ideation; approved for use in OCD and adolescent depression

 Pregnancy risk category C (some animal studies show adverse effects, no controlled studies in humans)

 Preliminary research suggests that it is safe for patients with cardiac impairment

 No dose adjustment for renal impairment; not removed by hemodialysis

 Lower dose by half or give less frequently for hepatic impairment

---

FIGURE 4.11. Dosing and safety information for fluoxetine.

Fluvoxamine

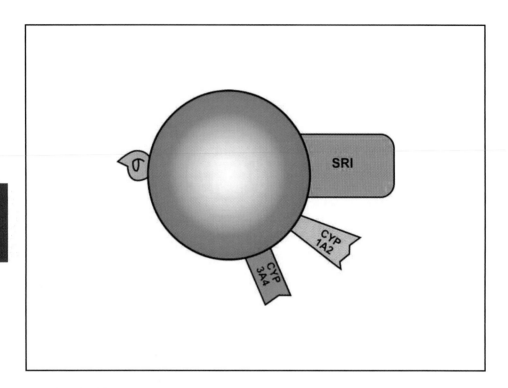

FIGURE 4.12. Fluvoxamine is approved to treat obsessive compulsive disorder and is used off-label to treat other disorders, including PTSD. Fluvoxamine has secondary actions at sigma 1 receptors (more potently than sertraline), which may contribute to increased anxiolytic efficacy. Fluvoxamine is also an inhibitor of both CYP450 3A4 and CYP450 1A2, and thus may have more drug interactions than other SSRIs.

Fluvoxamine: Tips and Pearls

Dosing and Use

Formulations:
IR tablets: 25 mg, 50 mg scored, 100 mg scored; CR capsules: 100 mg, 150 mg

Dosage Range:
100–300 mg/day for anxiety

Approved For:
Obsessive compulsive disorder, social anxiety disorder (controlled release formulation)

Side Effects and Safety

Weight Gain

unusual   not unusual   common   problematic

Sedation

unusual   not unusual   common   problematic

Rare: seizures, induction of mania, induction of suicidality in children, adolescents, and young adults

Do not use with MAOIs, thioridazine, pimozide, tizanidine, alosetron, ramelteon

Pearls

Often preferred treatment of anxious depression and comorbid major depression and anxiety disorders; sigma 1 actions may explain rapid onset effects in anxiety and insomnia; recently released in CR formulation

Special Populations

Use with caution in children; watch for activation of mania or suicidal ideation; approved for use in OCD

Pregnancy risk category C (some animal studies show adverse effects, no controlled studies in humans)

Preliminary research suggests it is safe for patients with cardiac impairment

No dose adjustment for renal impairment

Lower dose or give less frequently and use slower titration for hepatic impairment

FIGURE 4.13. Dosing and safety information for fluvoxamine.

Citalopram

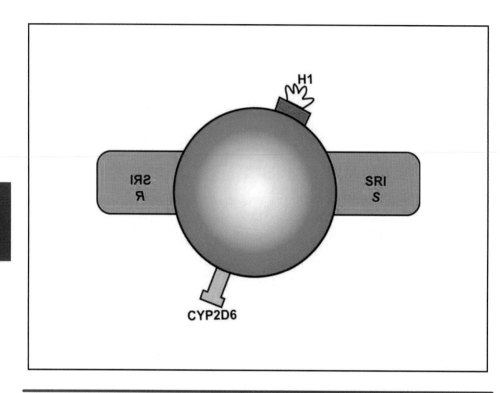

FIGURE 4.14. Citalopram is used off-label to treat multiple anxiety disorders, including PTSD. Citalopram consists of two enantiomers, R and S. Taken together, this agent is known as racemic citalopram, with mild antihistamine and CYP450 2D6 inhibitory properties residing in the R enantiomer. Citalopram may be somewhat inconsistent in therapeutic action at its lowest dose, potentially requiring a dose increase to optimize treatment response. This may be due to a recent finding that the R enantiomer may be active at the serotonin transporter (SERT), interfering with the ability of the S enantiomer to inhibit SERT. This interference could lead to reduced inhibition of SERT, reduced synaptic serotonin, and possibly reduced therapeutic action.

Citalopram: Tips and Pearls

<table>
<tr><td></td><td>Dosing and Use</td></tr>
</table>

Formulations:
Tablets 10 mg, 20 mg scored, 40 mg scored; orally disintegrating tablets: 10 mg, 20 mg, 40 mg; capsules: 10 mg, 20 mg, 40 mg

Dosage Range:
20–60 mg/day

Approved For:
Depression

Side Effects and Safety

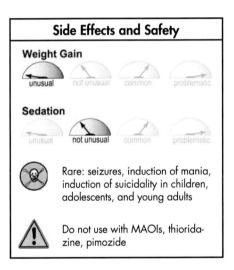

Weight Gain

unusual · not unusual · common · problematic

Sedation

unusual · not unusual · common · problematic

Rare: seizures, induction of mania, induction of suicidality in children, adolescents, and young adults

Do not use with MAOIs, thioridazine, pimozide

Pearls

 May be better tolerated than other SSRIs but less well tolerated than escitalopram; effective for comorbid depression

Special Populations

 Use with caution in children; watch for activation of mania or suicidal ideation

 Pregnancy risk category C (some animal studies show adverse effects, no controlled studies in humans)

 Preliminary research suggests it is safe for patients with cardiac impairment

 No dose adjustment for mild to moderate renal impairment; use with caution in severe impairment

 Recommended dose 20 mg/day for hepatic impairment; may raise to 40 mg/day in nonresponders

FIGURE 4.15. Dosing and safety information for citalopram.

Escitalopram

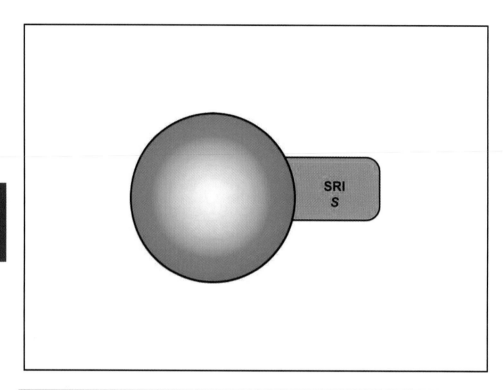

FIGURE 4.16. Escitalopram is approved to treat generalized anxiety disorder and is used off-label to treat PTSD. It is, in essence, citalopram with the R enantiomer removed, and thus lacks the antihistaminic and CYP450 2D6 inhibitory properties of citalopram, leaving the sole property of serotonin reuptake inhibition (SRI). Additionally, by removing the R enantiomer (which can interfere with SERT inhibition of the S enantiomer), the lowest dose of escitalopram may be more effective than the comparable dose of citalopram. Because of its truly selective mechanism of action, escitalopram has the lowest risk of drug interactions of all the SSRIs and may be the best tolerated as well.

Escitalopram: Tips and Pearls

 Dosing and Use

Formulations:
Tablets: 5 mg, 10 mg, 20 mg; capsules: 5 mg, 10 mg, 20 mg; liquid 5 mg/5 mL

Dosage Range:
10–20 mg/day

Approved For:
Generalized anxiety disorder, major depressive disorder

Side Effects and Safety

Weight Gain

unusual   not unusual   common   problematic

Sedation

unusual   not unusual   common   problematic

Rare: seizures, induction of mania, induction of suicidality in children, adolescents, and young adults

Do not use with MAOIs, pimozide

Pearls

May be among best-tolerated SSRIs due to its selective profile; effective for comorbid depression; commonly used with augmenting agents, as it has the least interaction at CYP450 2D6 and 3A4, causing fewer pharmacokinetically-mediated drug interactions

Special Populations

 Use with caution in children; watch for activation of mania or suicidal ideation; approved for use in adolescent depression

 Pregnancy risk category C (some animal studies show adverse effects, no controlled studies in humans)

 Not systematically evaluated in cardiac impairment, though citalopram safety may indicate safety of escitalopram

 No dose adjustment for mild to moderate renal impairment; use with caution in severe impairment

 Recommended dose 10 mg/day for hepatic impairment

FIGURE 4.17. Dosing and safety information for escitalopram.

Serotonin Norepinephrine Reuptake Inhibitors (SNRIs): Mechanism of Action

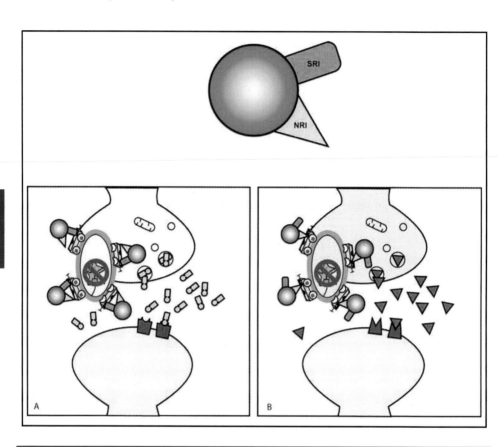

FIGURE 4.18. The SNRIs combine the serotonin reuptake inhibition (SRI) of SSRIs with norepinephrine reuptake inhibition (NRI). Thus they bind to the serotonin transporter, or SERT (A), and the norepinephrine transporter, or NET (B), preventing reuptake of serotonin and norepinephrine, respectively. As with the SSRIs, the underlying therapeutic mechanisms for SNRIs in PTSD are not known but are likely due to downstream effects (see Figures 4.3 and 4.4).

Of the SNRIs, only venlafaxine has been studied in controlled trials in PTSD; however, they are all included here as a first-line option due to their mechanistic similarity to venlafaxine and SSRIs as well as their evidence of efficacy in other anxiety disorders.

SNRIs

TABLE 4.2.	
Agent	**Approved in PTSD**
venlafaxine XR (Effexor XR, Efexor XR)	No
desvenlafaxine (Pristiq)	No
duloxetine (Cymbalta, Xeristar)	No
milnacipran (Savella, Ixel, Toledomin)	No

Venlafaxine

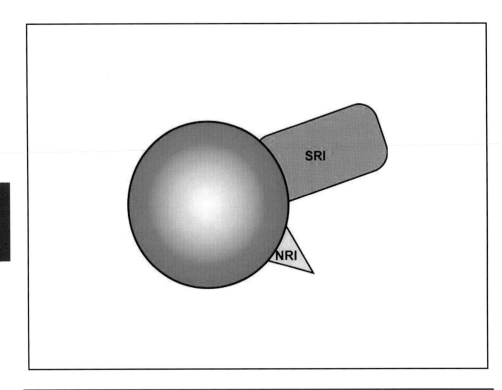

FIGURE 4.19. Venlafaxine is approved to treat multiple anxiety disorders, and has evidence of efficacy to treat PTSD. Venlafaxine's property of serotonin reuptake inhibition (SRI) is moderately potent and present at all doses, whereas its degree of norepinephrine reuptake inhibition (NRI) is dependent on dose (though even at high doses it is more serotonergic than noradrenergic). In addition, venlafaxine is converted to an active metabolite, desvenlafaxine, by CYP450 2D6. Desvenlafaxine has relatively more noradrenergic inhibition than the parent drug; thus noradrenergic activity may be even less with venlafaxine when given concomitantly with a CYP450 2D6 inhibitor. Discontinuation of venlafaxine may cause withdrawal reactions, especially after sudden discontinuation. The extended-release formulation is much better tolerated than the immediate-release formulation.

Venlafaxine: Tips and Pearls

 Dosing and Use

Formulations:
XR capsules: 37.5 mg, 75 mg, 150 mg; XR tablets: 37.5 mg, 75 mg, 150 mg, 225 mg; IR tablets: 25 mg scored, 37.5 mg scored, 50 mg scored, 75 mg scored, 100 mg scored

Dosage Range:
150–225 mg/day for anxiety (divided doses for immediate-release)

Approved For:
Generalized anxiety disorder, panic disorder, social anxiety disorder, depression

Side Effects and Safety

Weight Gain

unusual | not unusual | common | problematic

Sedation

unusual | not unusual | common | problematic

Rare: seizures, induction of mania, induction of suicidality in children, adolescents, and young adults

Do not use with MAOIs, uncontrolled narrow angle closure glaucoma

Pearls

 May be effective in a broad array of anxiety disorders; effective for co-morbid depression; greater potency for serotonin reuptake blockade than norepinephrine reuptake blockade but the clinical significance of this as a differentiating feature among SNRIs is unknown; efficacy and side effects are dose-dependent

Special Populations

 Use with caution in children; watch for activation of mania or suicidal ideation

 Pregnancy risk category C (some animal studies show adverse effects, no controlled studies in humans)

 Use with caution in patients with cardiac impairment; do not use in patients with uncontrolled hypertension; monitor blood pressure during treatment

 Lower dose by 25–50% for renal impairment; patients on dialysis should not receive subsequent dose until dialysis completed

 Lower dose by 50% for hepatic impairment

FIGURE 4.20. Dosing and safety information for venlafaxine.

Desvenlafaxine

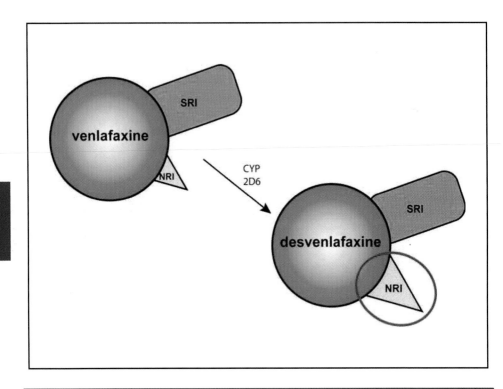

FIGURE 4.21. Desvenlafaxine, the active metabolite of venlafaxine, is not approved to treat any anxiety disorders but may be used off label. It is formed as a result of CYP450 2D6 but is not itself a substrate for any CYP450 enzyme; thus its plasma levels should be more consistent than those of venlafaxine. Although it is more potent at the serotonin transporter than at the norepinephrine transporter, it has greater norepinephrine reuptake inhibition (NRI) relative to serotonin reuptake inhibition (SRI) compared to venlafaxine.

Desvenlafaxine: Tips and Pearls

Dosing and Use

Formulations:
Tablets: 50 mg, 100 mg

Dosage Range:
50–100 mg/day; higher doses have been studied in depression

Approved For:
Major depressive disorder

Side Effects and Safety

Weight Gain

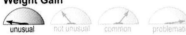

unusual · not unusual · common · problematic

Sedation

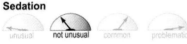

unusual · not unusual · common · problematic

 Rare: seizures, induction of mania, induction of suicidality in children, adolescents, and young adults

 Do not use with MAOIs, uncontrolled narrow angle closure glaucoma

Pearls

 Not specifically studied in anxiety disorders, though venlafaxine efficacy may indicate efficacy of desvenlafaxine; effective for comorbid depression; greater potency for norepinephrine reuptake blockade compared to venlafaxine but the clinical significance of this is unknown

Special Populations

 Use with caution in children; watch for activation of mania or suicidal ideation

 Pregnancy risk category C (some animal studies show adverse effects, no controlled studies in humans)

 Use with caution in patients with cardiac impairment; do not use in patients with uncontrolled hypertension; monitor blood pressure during treatment

 Recommended dose is 50 mg/day for moderate renal impairment and 50 mg every other day for severe impairment; patients on dialysis should not receive subsequent dose until dialysis completed

 Doses higher than 100 mg/day not recommended for hepatic impairment

FIGURE 4.22. Dosing and safety information for desvenlafaxine.

Duloxetine

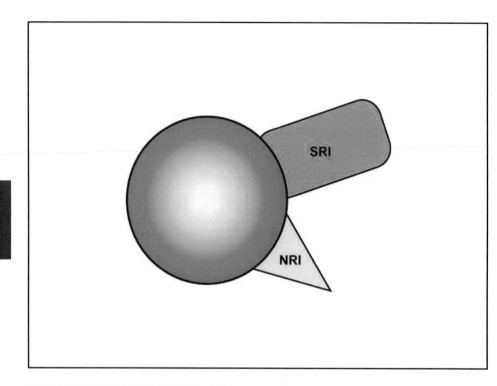

FIGURE 4.23. Duloxetine is approved to treat generalized anxiety disorder and is used but not approved to treat PTSD. Like venlafaxine and desvenlafaxine, duloxetine has greater serotonin reuptake inhibition (SRI) than norepinephrine reuptake inhibition (NRI); however, both serotonin and norepinephrine blockade may be present at the low end of the therapeutic dosing range. Duloxetine is a CYP450 2D6 inhibitor, which may result in various drug interactions that should be monitored.

Duloxetine: Tips and Pearls

Dosing and Use

Formulations:
Capsules: 20 mg, 30 mg, 60 mg

Dosage Range:
60 mg/day for anxiety; some patients may require 120 mg/day

Approved For:
Generalized anxiety disorder, major depressive disorder, diabetic peripheral neuropathic pain, fibromyalgia

Side Effects and Safety

Weight Gain

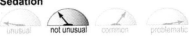

Sedation

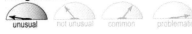

 Rare: seizures, induction of mania, induction of suicidality in children, adolescents, and young adults

 Do not use with MAOIs, thioridazine, uncontrolled narrow angle closure glaucoma, substantial alcohol use

Pearls

 Not well studied in anxiety other than generalized anxiety disorder, but likely effective; effective for comorbid depression; only somewhat greater potency for serotonin reuptake blockade than norepinephrine reuptake blockade but the clinical significance of this as a differentiating feature among SNRIs is unknown

Special Populations

 Use with caution in children; watch for activation of mania or suicidal ideation

 Pregnancy risk category C (some animal studies show adverse effects, no controlled studies in humans)

 Use with caution in patients with cardiac impairment; may raise blood pressure

 Not recommended for use in patients with end-stage renal disease or severe renal impairment

 Not to be used in patients with any hepatic insufficiency; not recommended for use in patients with substantial alcohol use

FIGURE 4.24. Dosing and safety information for duloxetine.

Milnacipran

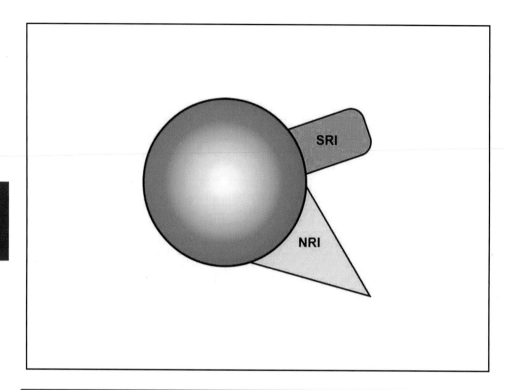

FIGURE 4.25. Milnacipran is neither approved nor widely used to treat anxiety disorders. It is somewhat different than other SNRIs in that it has the strongest norepinephrine reuptake inhibition (NRI) relative to serotonin reuptake inhibition (SRI) among the four approved agents. Some data even suggest that its actions at the norepinephrine transporter are stronger than those at the serotonin transporter, while the other SNRIs are generally the opposite. Milnacipran may be more energizing and activating than some other SNRIs due to its relatively potent noradrenergic actions, which could be disadvantageous for patients with anxiety, at least in the short term.

Milnacipran: Tips and Pearls

Dosing and Use

Formulations:
Capsules (not in U.S): 15 mg, 25 mg, 50 mg; tablets (U.S.): 12.5 mg, 25 mg, 50 mg, 100 mg

Dosage Range:
30–200 mg/day in 2 doses

Approved For:
Fibromyalgia

Pearls

Not specifically studied in anxiety disorders; effective for comorbid depression; greater potency for norepinephrine reuptake blockade than serotonin reuptake blockade but the clinical significance of this as a differentiating feature among SNRIs is unknown; potent noradrenergic actions may account for higher incidence of sweating and urinary hesitancy as well as theoretical advantages for cognitive symptoms

Side Effects and Safety

Weight Gain

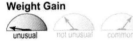
unusual · not unusual · common · problematic

Sedation

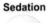
unusual · not unusual · common · problematic

Rare: seizures, induction of mania, induction of suicidality in children, adolescents, and young adults

Do not use with MAOIs, uncontrolled narrow angle closure glaucoma

Special Populations

Use with caution in children; watch for activation of mania or suicidal ideation

Pregnancy risk category C (some animal studies show adverse effects, no controlled studies in humans)

Use with caution in patients with cardiac impairment

Use with caution in patients with moderate renal impairment; recommended dose 50–100 mg/day for severe impairment

No dose adjustment necessary for hepatic impairment; not recommended for use in chronic liver disease

FIGURE 4.26. Dosing and safety information for milnacipran.

Second-Line, Adjunct, and Investigational Medications for PTSD

In addition to the first-line selective serotonin reuptake inhibitors (SSRIs) and serotonin norepinephrine reuptake inhibitors (SNRIs), there are many second-line and adjunct pharmacologic options for PTSD. In this chapter, the mechanisms of action of such agents are explained and clinical characteristics are briefly reviewed. Several agents under investigation for their potential use in PTSD are reviewed as well.

SECTION ONE
Second-line Medications

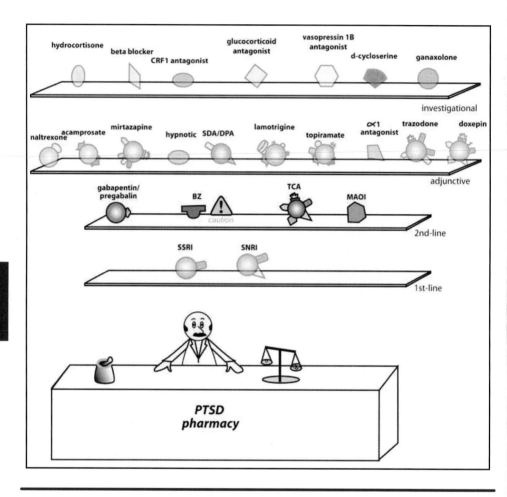

FIGURE 5.1. Second-line medications for PTSD include tricyclic antidepressants (TCAs); monoamine oxidase inhibitors (MAOIs); the alpha 2 delta ligands, gabapentin and pregabalin; and anxiolytic benzodiazepines.

Tricyclic Antidepressants (TCAs):
Mechanism of Action

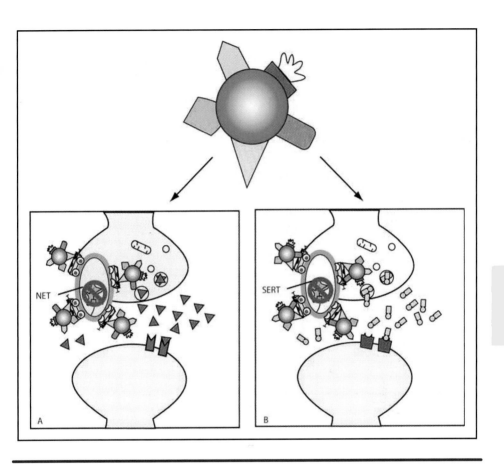

FIGURE 5.2. Like the SNRIs, the primary mechanisms of action for tricyclic antidepressants (TCAs) are blockade of the serotonin transporter, or SERT (B), and the norepinephrine transporter, or NET (A), preventing reuptake of serotonin and norepinephrine, respectively. Some TCAs are more selective for serotonergic mechanisms and some are more strongly noradrenergic, although all TCAs block reuptake of both neurotransmitters to some extent.

The TCA Family

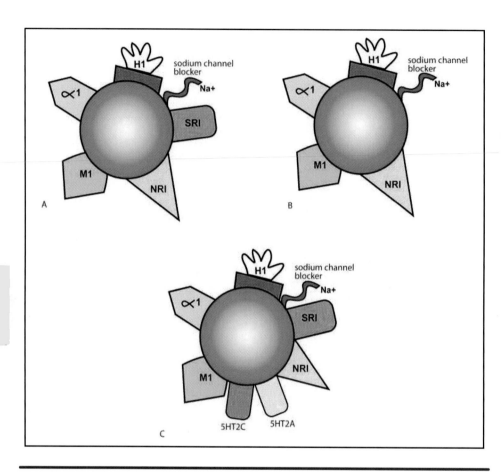

FIGURE 5.3. TCAs, although considered as efficacious as the SSRIs and SNRIs for depression, have several unwanted mechanisms that contribute to a worse tolerability profile. Histamine H1 receptor blockade may relieve insomnia but can also cause sedation and may lead to weight gain. Muscarinic M1 receptor blockade causes dry mouth, blurred vision, urinary retention, and constipation, while muscarinic M3 receptor blockade can interfere with insulin action. Alpha 1 adrenergic receptor blockade causes orthostatic hypotension and dizziness. In very high doses, TCAs' weak blockade of voltage-sensitive sodium channels in the heart and brain is thought to be the cause of coma and seizures.

Selections from the TCA Family

Amitriptyline
Elavil

Dosage Range:
50–150 mg/day

Approved For:
Depression

Pearls:
Stronger serotonergic action; significant drug-drug interactions; use with caution in patients with renal, hepatic, or cardiac impairment; can have cardiovascular effects and should not be used in some patients; pregnancy risk category C

Imipramine
Tofranil

Dosage Range:
50–150 mg/day

Approved For:
Depression

Pearls:
Stronger serotonergic action; significant drug-drug interactions; use with caution in patients with renal, hepatic, or cardiac impairment; can have cardiovascular effects and should not be used in some patients; pregnancy risk category D

Desipramine
Norpramin

Dosage Range:
100–200 mg/day

Approved For:
Depression

Pearls:
Stronger noradrenergic action; may have lower rate of anticholinergic and hypotensive effects than other TCAs; significant drug-drug interactions; use with caution in patients with renal, hepatic, or cardiac impairment; can have cardiovascular effects and should not be used in some patients; pregnancy risk category C

Nortriptyline
Pamelor

Dosage Range:
50–150 mg/day

Approved For:
Major depressive disorder

Pearls:
Stronger noradrenergic action; may have lower rate of anticholinergic and hypotensive effects than other TCAs; significant drug-drug interactions; use with caution in patients with renal, hepatic, or cardiac impairment; can have cardiovascular effects and should not be used in some patients; pregnancy risk category D

FIGURE 5.4. Brief clinical characteristics of select TCAs prescribed for PTSD.

Monoamine Oxidase Inhibitors (MAOIs):
Mechanism of Action

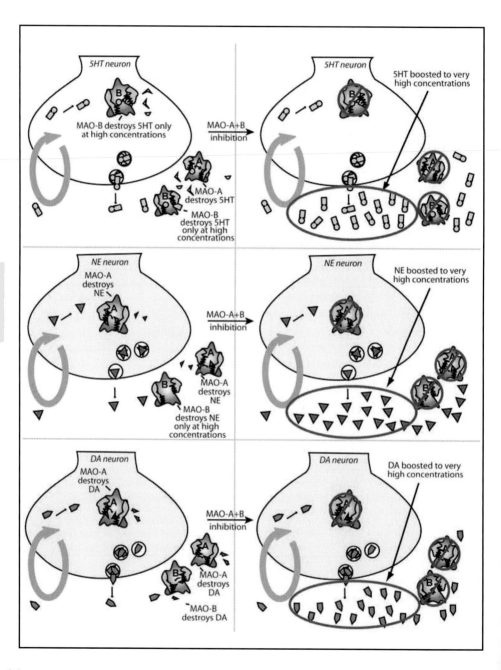

Monoamine Oxidase Inhibitors (MAOIs):
Mechanism of Action (cont.)

FIGURE 5.5. The enzyme monoamine oxidase A (MAO-A) metabolizes serotonin (5HT), norepinephrine (NE), and dopamine (DA) (left panels). Monoamine oxidase B (MAO-B) also metabolizes DA, but it metabolizes 5HT and NE only at high concentrations (left panels). Thus inhibition of MAO-A increases 5HT and NE but has little effect on DA (because MAO-B is still able to metabolize it). In contrast, inhibition of MAO-B does not have great effect on 5HT or NE, but does increase DA to some extent (though MAO-A is still available to metabolize it). Combined inhibition of MAO-A and MAO-B leads to greater increases in each of these neurotransmitters than inhibition of either enzyme alone (right panels).

MAOIs, Tyramine, and Hypertensive Crisis

A. Hypertensive Crisis

Defined as diastolic blood pressure > 120 mmHg

Symptoms include: occipital headache that may radiate frontally, palpitation, neck stiffness or soreness, nausea, vomiting, sweating (sometimes with fever), dilated pupils, photophobia, tachycardia or bradycardia that can be associated with constricting chest pain

B. Dietary Modifications for Patients on MAO Inhibitors*

Foods to Avoid	Foods Allowed
Dried, aged, smoked, fermented, spoiled, or improperly stored meat, poultry, or fish	Fresh or processed meat, poultry, or fish
Broad bean pods	All other vegetables
Aged cheeses	Processed and cottage cheese, ricotta cheese, yogurt
Tap and nonpasteurized beers	Canned or bottled beers and alcohol
Marmite, sauerkraut	Brewer's and baker's yeast
Soy products, tofu	

*No dietary modifications needed for low doses of transdermal or oral selective MAO-B inhibitors.

TABLE 5.1. Tyramine, an amine present in various foods including cheese, acts to increase release of norepinephrine. A meal high in tyramine (40 mg or more), combined with inhibition of MAO-A (which also increases norepinephrine) can lead to a high accumulation of norepinephrine and potentially dangerous vasoconstriction and hypertension. In some cases this can lead to hypertensive crisis, a potentially fatal reaction (see characteristics in part A). The risk can be controlled by restricting tyramine intake (see dietary suggestions in part B).

Drugs to Avoid with MAOIs

C. Drugs to Avoid for Patients on MAO Inhibitors Due to Risk of Hypertensive Crisis

<u>Decongestants</u>: phenylephrine, ephedrine (ma huang, ephedra), pseudoephedrine, phenyl-propanolamine

<u>Stimulants</u>: amphetamines, methylphenidate

<u>Antidepressants</u>: TCAs, atomoxetine, reboxetine, venlafaxine, desvenlafaxine, duloxetine, milnacipran, bupropion

<u>Appetite suppressants</u>: sibutramine, phentermine

D. Drugs Contraindicated in Combination with MAO Inhibitors Due to Risk of Serotonin Syndrome

<u>Antidepressants</u>: fluoxetine, fluvoxamine, paroxetine, sertraline, citalopram, escitalopram, venlafaxine, desvenlafaxine, duloxetine, milnacipran, TCAs (especially clomipramine)

<u>Other TCA structures</u>: cyclobenzapine, carbamazepine

<u>Appetite suppressants</u>: sibutramine

<u>Opioids</u>: dextromethorphan, meperidine, tramadol, methadone, propoxyphene

TABLE 5.2. Some drugs with noradrenergic actions can also lead to hypertensive crisis when combined with MAOIs and should be avoided (A).

Combination of MAOIs with agents that inhibit serotonin reuptake can also be dangerous, as combining two different methods of increasing serotonin may lead to a dramatic accumulation of serotonin. This can cause excessive stimulation of postsynaptic serotonin receptors and lead to hyperthermia, coma, seizures, cardio-vascular problems, and death. This is known as the "serotonin syndrome" and is why the combination of an MAOI with any drug that has SRI properties is strictly contraindicated (B).

MAOIs with Reduced Risk
of Tyramine Reactions

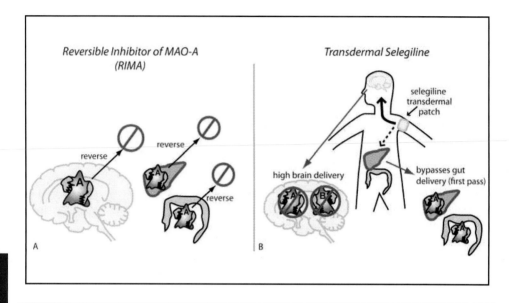

FIGURE 5.6. MAOIs presumably must inhibit MAO-A in the brain for therapeutic effects in anxiety disorders. However, they also cause simultaneous inhibition of MAO-A in the liver and intestinal mucosa, which creates risk of tyramine reactions.

(A) One mechanism for preserving the effects in the brain while avoiding effects in the gut is reversible inhibition of MAO-A (RIMA). RIMAs can be removed from the enzyme by competitors (e.g., norepinephrine). Thus the accumulation of norepinephrine released by tyramine can displace the RIMA, allowing norepinephrine to be destroyed and reducing risk of a tyramine reaction.

(B) A second way to combat this dilemma is with transdermal selegiline. The selective MAO-B inhibitor must be administered in high doses in order to inhibit MAO-A as well. Transdermal administration of selegiline delivers the drug directly into the systemic circulation, hitting the brain in high doses but avoiding a first pass through the liver and thus reducing risk of a tyramine reaction.

Selections from the MAOI Family

Moclobemide
Aurorix, Arima, Manerix

Dosage Range:
300–600 mg/day in 3 doses

Approved For:
Not approved in United States

Pearls:
Reversible, selective inhibitor of MAO-A; approved in other countries for depression and social anxiety disorder; requires food restrictions but has reduced risk of tyramine reactions compared to irreversible, nonselective MAOIs; many significant drug-drug interactions and contraindications; use with caution in patients with renal impairment; may require lower dose in patients with hepatic or cardiac impairment; not generally recommended during pregnancy

Phenelzine
Nardil, Nardelzine

Dosage Range:
45–75 mg/day in 3 doses

Approved For:
Depressed patients characterized as "atypical," "nonendogenous," or "neurotic"

Pearls:
Irreversible, nonselective MAO inhibitor; requires food restrictions; many significant drug-drug interactions and contraindications; may require lower dose in patients with renal impairment; contraindicated in patients with hepatic impairment, congestive heart failure, or hypertension; may require lower dose for other cardiac impairment; pregnancy risk category C

Selegiline
EMSAM (transdermal)

Dosage Range:
6–12 mg/24 hours

Approved For:
Major depressive disorder

Pearls:
MAO-A and B inhibitor in the brain and relatively selective MAO-B inhibitor in the gut; food restrictions only at high doses (30 mg/24 hours or higher); many significant drug-drug interactions and contraindications; metabolized to amphetamine; may require lower dose in patients with cardiac impairment; pregnancy risk category C

Tranylcypromine
Parnate

Dosage Range:
30 mg/day in divided doses

Approved For:
Major depressive episode without melancholia

Pearls:
Irreversible, nonselective MAO inhibitor; better studied in panic disorder than in PTSD but not approved for either; requires food restrictions; many significant drug-drug interactions and contraindications; has amphetamine-like properties; may require lower dose in patients with renal impairment; contraindicated in patients with hepatic or cardiac impairment, pregnancy risk category C

FIGURE 5.7. Brief clinical characteristics of select MAOIs prescribed for PTSD.

Alpha 2 Delta Ligands:
Mechanism of Action

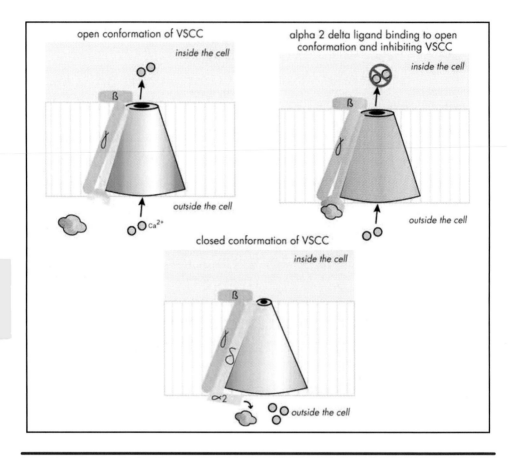

FIGURE 5.8. The role of voltage-sensitive calcium channels (VSCCs) in regulating neurotransmission was illustrated in Figure 3.15. Pathological anxiety and fear may be caused by overactivation of amygdala circuits; thus modulating VSCC activity within those circuits may normalize neurotransmission and reduce symptoms.

Alpha 2 delta ligands bind selectively to VSCCs and actually appear to bind with higher affinity to VSCCs in the open channel conformation. Thus they may exert greater effects in situations where neurons have excessive activity, as hypothesized for amygdala circuits in anxiety disorders, while not interfering with normal neurotransmission in neurons uninvolved in mediating the pathological anxiety state.

Alpha 2 Delta Ligands:
Gabapentin and Pregabalin

 Gabapentin
Neurontin

Dosage Range:
900–1800 mg/day in 2 or 3 doses

Approved For:
Partial seizures, postherpetic neuralgia

Pearls:
Not studied in PTSD but evidence of efficacy in social anxiety and panic disorders; well tolerated with only mild side effects; most use is off-label; enhances slow-wave delta sleep; approved in children for seizures (adjunct); pregnancy risk category C

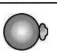 **Pregabalin**
Lyrica

Dosage Range:
150–600 mg/day in 2 or 3 doses

Approved For:
Partial seizures (adjunct), fibromyalgia, diabetic peripheral neuropathic pain, postherpetic neuralgia

Pearls:
Not studied in PTSD but approved in Europe for anxiety disorders; well tolerated with only mild side effects; few pharmacokinetic interactions; enhances slow-wave delta sleep; do not use in patients with a problem of galactose intolerance, the Lapp lactase deficiency, or glucose-galactose malabsorption; pregnancy risk category C

FIGURE 5.9. Brief clinical characteristics of alpha 2 delta ligands.

Benzodiazepines:
Mechanism of Action

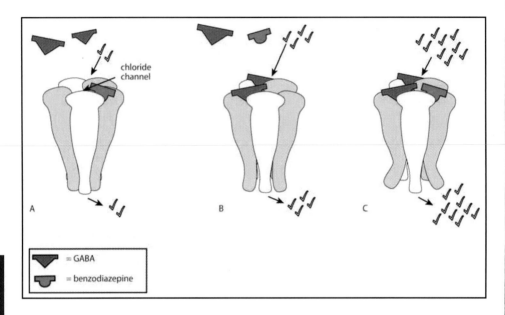

FIGURE 5.10. GABA is the major inhibitory neurotransmitter in the brain and has multiple receptors (Figures 3.11 and 3.12). Benzodiazepines exert their anxiolytic actions at GABA-A receptors, as illustrated here.

GABA-A receptors consist of five subunits with a central chloride channel and have binding sites not only for GABA but also for benzodiazepines. When a benzodiazepine binds to the GABA-A receptor in the absence of GABA it has no effect on the GABA channel—chloride conductance is the same as in the resting state (A). When GABA binds to its site on the GABA-A receptor, it increases the frequency of opening of the chloride channel, allowing more chloride to pass through (B). When a benzodiazepine binds to the GABA-A receptor in the presence of GABA it causes the channel to open even more frequently than when GABA alone is present (C). This type of mechanism is termed positive allosteric modulation.

Selections from the Benzodiazepine Family

 Alprazolam
Xanax

Dosage Range:
IR 1–6 mg/day in 3 doses; XR 3–6 mg/day

Approved For:
Generalized anxiety disorder, panic disorder

Pearls:
Lack of evidence of efficacy in PTSD; use caution as many patients with PTSD may have substance abuse; use with caution in patients with renal impairment; use lower dose for patients with hepatic impairment and in the elderly; do not use with ketoconazole or itraconazole; do not use if patient has narrow angle-closure glaucoma; pregnancy risk category D

 Clonazepam
Klonopin

Dosage Range:
0.5–2 mg/day

Approved For:
Panic disorder, various seizure disorders

Pearls:
Lack of evidence of efficacy in PTSD; use caution as many patients with PTSD may have substance abuse; use lower dose for patients with renal or mild/moderate hepatic impairment and in the elderly; do not use if patient has narrow angle-closure glaucoma or severe liver disease; pregnancy risk category D

 Diazepam
Valium, Diastat

Dosage Range:
4–40 mg/day in 2–4 doses

Approved For:
Oral: anxiety disorder, acute alcohol withdrawal symptoms, spasticity, athetosis, Stiffman syndrome, convulsive disorder (adjunct)

Pearls:
Lack of evidence of efficacy in PTSD; use caution as many patients with PTSD may have substance abuse; use lower dose for patients with renal or hepatic impairment and in the elderly; do not use if patient has narrow angle-closure glaucoma; pregnancy risk category D

 Lorazepam
Ativan

Dosage Range:
2–6 mg/day in 2–3 doses

Approved For:
Oral: anxiety disorder, anxiety associated with depressive symptoms

Pearls:
Lack of evidence of efficacy in PTSD; use caution as many patients with PTSD may have substance abuse; use lower dose for patients with renal or hepatic impairment and in the elderly; do not use if patient has narrow angle-closure glaucoma; pregnancy risk category D

FIGURE 5.11. Brief clinical characteristics of anxiolytic benzodiazepines.

SECTION TWO
Adjunct Medications

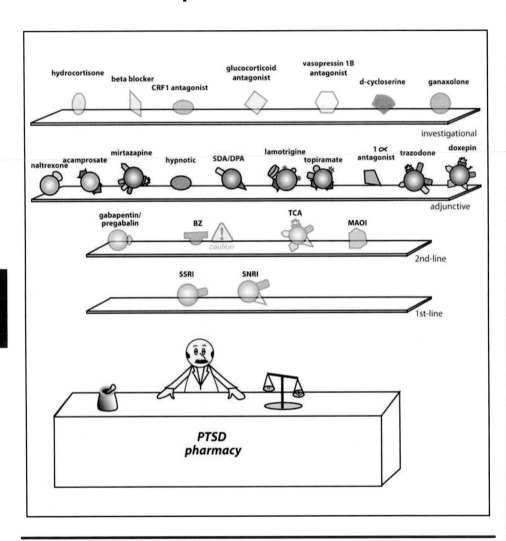

FIGURE 5.12. Adjunct medications for PTSD include agents that may treat residual anxiety (e.g., mirtazapine, atypical antipsychotics) as well as those that target specific symptoms (e.g., alpha 1 antagonists for nightmares, sedative hypnotics for sleep disturbances) or comorbidities (e.g., naltrexone and acamprosate for alcohol abuse/dependence).

Sedating Antidepressants, Part 1

Mirtazapine
Remeron

Dosage Range:
15–45 mg/night

Approved For:
Major depressive disorder

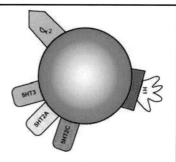

Pearls:
Preliminary evidence of efficacy in PTSD as monotherapy and as adjunct; weight gain can be common; sedation can be common; hypnotic properties can be desirable for states of hyper-arousal and especially at night; few pharmacokinetic interactions; use with caution in patients with renal or cardiac impairment; use lower dose for patients with hepatic impairment; do not use with MAO inhibitors; pregnancy risk category C

FIGURE 5.13. Mirtazapine has multiple mechanisms that may contribute to its thera-peutic profile. It has actions at alpha 2 receptors as well as three 5HT receptors— 2A, 2C, and 3—and also blocks histamine 1 (H1) receptors.

By blocking alpha 2 receptors, mirtazapine increases both serotonin and norepi-nephrine; however, because 5HT2A, 2C, and 3 receptors are also blocked by mir-tazapine, the net stimulation falls on 5HT1A receptors. This further results in release of dopamine, which may be helpful in depression as well as anxiety. Mirtazapine's antagonist actions at 5HT2A and 2C receptors also result in increased release of dopamine and norepinephrine, which may contribute to anxiolytic, antidepressant, and sleep-restoring properties. Finally, H1 receptor antagonism may help relieve insomnia and anxiety but may also cause sedation and contribute to weight gain.

Sedating Antidepressants, Part 2

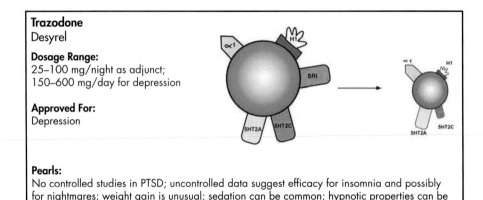

Trazodone
Desyrel

Dosage Range:
25–100 mg/night as adjunct;
150–600 mg/day for depression

Approved For:
Depression

Pearls:
No controlled studies in PTSD; uncontrolled data suggest efficacy for insomnia and possibly for nightmares; weight gain is unusual; sedation can be common; hypnotic properties can be desirable for states of hyperarousal and especially at night; use with caution in patients with hepatic or cardiac impairment; do not use with MAO inhibitors; pregnancy risk category C

FIGURE 5.14. At antidepressant doses (150–600 mg/day), trazodone is a potent antagonist at serotonin 2A receptors and also blocks serotonin 2C receptors and the serotonin transporter. In addition, its blockade of histamine 1 receptors is largely responsible for its sedative effects, while blockade of alpha 1 adrenergic receptors may contribute to efficacy for treating nightmares (see Figure 5.16). At low doses (25–100 mg/night), trazodone does not adequately block serotonin reuptake but does retain its other properties and thus can still be sedating.

Sedating Antidepressants, Part 3

Doxepin
Sinequan

Dosage Range:
1–6 mg/night for insomnia;
150–300 mg/day for depression

Approved For:
Psychoneurotic patient with depression
and/or anxiety; depression and/or
anxiety associated with alcoholism or
with organic disease; psychotic depressive disorders with associated anxiety;
involutional depression; manic depressive
disorder

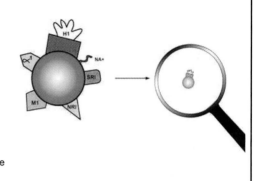

Pearls:
Not studied in PTSD; may be useful at low doses (requires liquid formulation) as an adjunct for
insomnia; weight gain can be common; sedation can be common; hypnotic properties can be
desirable for states of hyperarousal and especially at night; significant drug-drug interactions at
antidepressant doses; use with caution in patients with renal or hepatic impairment; can have
cardiovascular effects and should not be used in some patients; do not use with MAO inhibitors; do not use in patients with narrow angle-closure glaucoma; pregnancy risk category C

FIGURE 5.15. Doxepin is a tricyclic antidepressant that, at antidepressant doses
(150–300 mg/day) inhibits serotonin and norepinephrine reuptake and is an antagonist at histamine 1, muscarine 1, and alpha 1 adrenergic receptors. At low
doses (1–6 mg/night), however, doxepin is quite selective for histamine 1 receptors
and thus may be used as a hypnotic.

Alpha 1 Antagonists for Nightmares

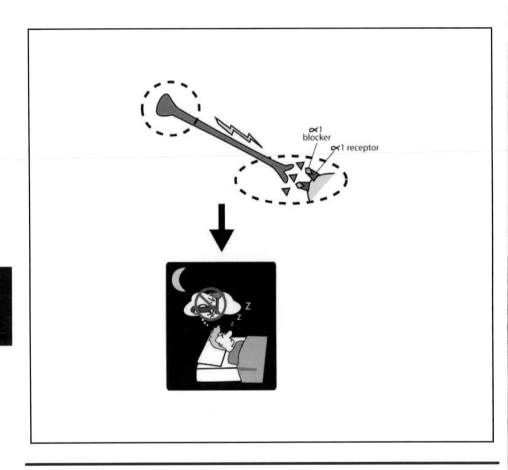

FIGURE 5.16. Noradrenergic neurons (Figure 3.7) originate in the locus coeruleus, which is responsible for the autonomic output of fear (Figure 1.4), and innervate the amygdala and the prefrontal cortex, both of which are essential to anxiety and worry (Figures 1.2 through 1.8). Alpha adrenergic blockers may modulate the anxiogenic effects of noradrenergic hyperactivation (see Figure 3.8). Interestingly, alpha adrenergic receptors are also involved in sleep responses, and may thus be relevant to the sleep disturbances and nightmares associated with PTSD.

Prazosin, an alpha 1 adrenergic blocker approved for the treatment of hypertension, has been used to prevent nightmares in patients with PTSD. Such use has not been extensively studied, but early clinical data suggest that it may be efficacious.

Sedative Hypnotics

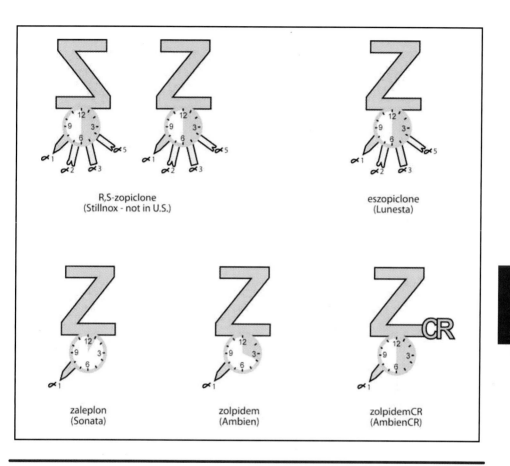

FIGURE 5.17. Sleep disturbances are common in patients with PTSD. Implementing good sleep hygiene techniques is important for these patients; in addition, the use of sedative hypnotics may be beneficial. Zaleplon, zolpidem, zopiclone, and eszopiclone bind to GABA-A receptors, as do the benzodiazepines (Figures 5.10 and 5.11), but they do so in a way that does not generally cause tolerance, dependence, or withdrawal upon discontinuation. Zaleplon and zolpidem are also selective for GABA-A receptors containing the alpha 1 subtype, which theoretically could contribute to the lower risk of tolerance and dependence with these agents. However, these agents may need to be restricted in PTSD due to the frequent association of comorbid alcohol and drug abuse.

Adjunct Medications for Sleep-Related Problems

Prazosin
Minipress

Dosage Range:
1–20 mg/day

Approved For:
Hypertension

Pearls:
Early clinical data suggest it may be efficacious for preventing nightmares; weight gain is unusual; sedation is not unusual; most common side effects are dizziness and lightheadedness; syncope with sudden loss of consciousness can occur; pregnancy risk category C

Zaleplon
Sonata

Dosage Range:
10 mg at bedtime for 7–10 days

Approved For:
Short-term treatment of insomnia

Pearls:
Best for patients with trouble falling asleep; weight gain is unusual; sedation is common; use with caution in patients with severe renal impairment; use lower dose for patients with mild to moderate hepatic impairment and in the elderly, not recommended for patients with severe hepatic impairment; pregnancy risk category C

Zolpidem
Ambien

Dosage Range:
IR 10 mg at bedtime for 7–10 days; CR 12.5 mg/day at bedtime

Approved For:
Insomnia (IR indication is restricted to short-term)

Pearls:
Targets time to sleep onset, total sleep time, and nighttime awakenings; weight gain is unusual; sedation is common; use with caution in patients with renal impairment; use lower dose for patients with hepatic impairment and in the elderly; pregnancy risk category B

Eszopiclone
Lunesta

Dosage Range:
2–3 mg at bedtime

Approved For:
Insomnia

Pearls:
Targets time to sleep onset, total sleep time, and nighttime awakenings; weight gain is unusual; sedation is common; use lower dose for patients with severe hepatic impairment and in the elderly; pregnancy risk category C

FIGURE 5.18. Brief clinical characteristics of some adjunct medications prescribed for sleep-related problems.

Atypical Antipsychotics

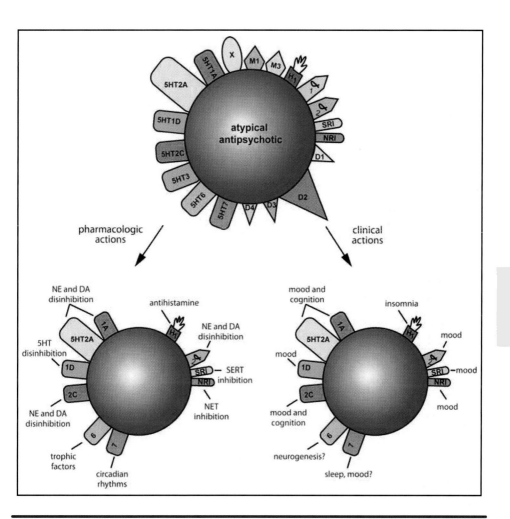

FIGURE 5.19. Atypical antipsychotics are best known as treatments of psychosis in schizophrenia and acute mania in bipolar disorder. However, these agents are increasingly being used to treat other disorders as well, including depression and anxiety disorders. Pharmacologically this makes sense, as their shared mechanisms—serotonin 2A antagonism and dopamine 2 antagonism/partial agonism—lead to modulation of the serotonin and dopamine systems. In addition, each agent has a unique secondary profile (see above and Figures 5.20 through 5.27) that may further contribute to therapeutic actions in various disorders.

Risperidone

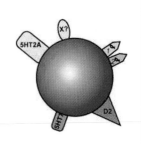

Risperidone
Risperdal

Dosage Range:
2–8 mg/day

Approved For:
Schizophrenia, ages 13 and older; delaying relapse in schizophrenia; other psychotic disorders; acute mania/mixed mania, ages 10 and older (monotherapy and adjunct); bipolar maintenance (CONSTA, monotherapy and adjunct), autism-related irritability, ages 5–16

Pearls:
Preliminary evidence of efficacy in PTSD as adjunct; commonly prescribed for aggression, agitation, and irritability associated with other disorders; most frequently used atypical antipsychotic in children and adolescents; weight gain and sedation can be common; dose-dependent extrapyramidal side effects (EPS) and prolactin elevation; use lower dose for patients with renal or hepatic impairment; use with caution in patients with cardiac impairment and in the elderly; pregnancy risk category C

FIGURE 5.20. In addition to being a serotonin 2A/dopamine 2 antagonist, risperidone blocks alpha 2 adrenergic receptors, which may contribute to efficacy for depression. It also blocks alpha 1 adrenergic receptors, which may contribute to orthostatic hypotension and sedation but could also potentially be therapeutic for sleep disturbances in PTSD (see Figure 5.16). Receptor "X" in the icon above represents the unclear actions that some atypical antipsychotics have on the insulin system, where they change cellular insulin resistance and increase fasting plasma triglyceride levels.

Olanzapine

Olanzapine
Zyprexa

Dosage Range:
10–20 mg/day

Approved For:
Oral: schizophrenia, ages 13 and older; maintaining response in schizophrenia; acute mania/mixed mania, ages 13 and older (monotherapy and adjunct); bipolar maintenance; bipolar depression (in combination with fluoxetine); treatment-resistant depression (in combination with fluoxetine)

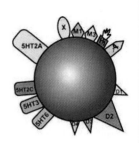

Pearls:
Preliminary evidence of efficacy in PTSD as adjunct; weight gain can be common and problematic; sedation can be common; use lower dose for patients with hepatic impairment; use with caution in patients with cardiac impairment and in the elderly; pregnancy risk category C

FIGURE 5.21. Olanzapine has widespread actions on the serotonin and dopamine systems and also blocks muscarinic 1 and 3 receptors, alpha adrenergic 1 receptors, and histamine 1 receptors. 5HT2C blockade may contribute to antidepressant effects and improve cognitive problems, but may also (potentially in concert with H1 antagonism) contribute to weight gain. Histamine 1, alpha 1 adrenergic, and muscarinic 1 receptor antagonism can cause sedation. Receptor "X" in the icon above represents the unclear actions that some atypical antipsychotics have on the insulin system, where they change cellular insulin resistance and increase fasting plasma triglyceride levels.

Quetiapine

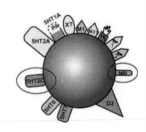

Quetiapine
Seroquel

Dosage Range:
300–800 mg/day

Approved For:
Acute schizophrenia, ages 13 and older; schizophrenia maintenance; acute mania, ages 10 and older (monotherapy and adjunct); bipolar maintenance; bipolar depression; treatment-resistant depression (adjunct)

Pearls:
Perhaps the most widely used antipsychotic agent in PSTD despite no controlled studies in PTSD as adjunct; weight gain can be common; sedation can be common and may not be tolerable, although hypnotic properties are often desirable for states of hyperarousal and especially at night; may need to use lower dose for patients with hepatic impairment; use with caution in patients with cardiac impairment; use with caution in the elderly and may need to lower dose; pregnancy risk category C

FIGURE 5.22. Quetiapine has widespread actions on the serotonin and dopamine systems and also blocks muscarinic 1 and 3 receptors, alpha adrenergic 1 and 2 receptors, and histamine 1 receptors. Its active metabolite, norquetiapine, has unique features (red circles) that most likely add to quetiapine's efficacy. The partial 5HT1A agonist feature of quetiapine and the 5HT2C antagonism and norepinephrine reuptake inhibition of norquetiapine are hypothetically responsible for its antidepressant and pro-cognitive effects. Alpha 2 adrenergic antagonism may also be a factor in antidepressant effects. 5HT2C blockade may contribute to weight gain, particularly in association with H1 blockade. Histamine 1, alpha 1 adrenergic, and muscarinic 1 receptor antagonism can cause sedation, though H1 blockade may also improve sleep disturbances. Receptor "X" in the icon above represents the unclear actions that some atypical antipsychotics have on the insulin system, where they change cellular insulin resistance and increase fasting plasma triglyceride levels.

Aripiprazole

Aripiprazole
Abilify

Dosage Range:
2–30 mg/day

Approved For:
Schizophrenia, ages 13 and older; maintaining stability in
schizophrenia; acute mania/mixed mania, ages 10 and
older; bipolar maintenance; depression (adjunct); irritability
in autism, ages 6 to 17

Pearls:
No controlled studies in PTSD as adjunct; weight gain and sedation are not common; can be
activating; use with caution in patients with cardiac impairment and in the elderly; pregnancy risk category C

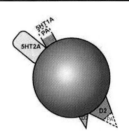

FIGURE 5.23. Aripiprazole functions primarily as a dopamine 2 partial agonist and
is also a 5HT2A antagonist. In addition, it is a 5HT1A partial agonist, which may
contribute to antidepressant and pro-cognitive effects. The clinical significance of
its D3 partial agonist property is unknown, but it theoretically may contribute to
antidepressant effects.

Ziprasidone

Ziprasidone
Geodon

Dosage Range:
80–160 mg/day in divided doses

Approved For:
Oral: schizophrenia; delaying relapse in schizophrenia;
acute mania/mixed mania; bipolar maintenance

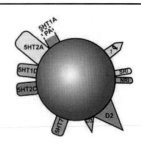

Pearls:
Not studied in PTSD but evidence of efficacy in other anxiety disorders; weight gain and
sedation are not common; can be activating, especially at low doses; do not use in patients
taking QTc-prolonging agents or in those with known history of QTc prolongation, recent
acute myocardial infarction, or uncompensated heart failure; use with caution in patients
with other cardiac impairment and in the elderly; pregnancy risk category C

FIGURE 5.24. Ziprasidone has actions on the serotonin, dopamine, and norepinephrine systems. Its 5HT1D and 5HT2C antagonism as well as serotonin and norepinephrine reuptake blocking properties could contribute to potential antidepressant
and anxiolytic effects, and 5HT2C antagonism may enhance cognition as well.
At high doses, alpha 1 adrenergic antagonism could contribute to sedation and
hypotension.

Paliperidone

Paliperidone
Invega

Dosage Range:
6 mg/day

Approved For:
Schizophrenia, maintaining response in schizophrenia,
schizoaffective disorder

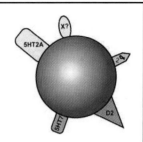

Pearls:
Not studied in PTSD but rationale for use based on preliminary evidence of efficacy for
risperidone as adjunct; weight gain and sedation can be common; dose-dependent extrapyramidal side effects (EPS) and prolactin elevation; use lower dose for patients with renal
impairment; use with caution in patients with cardiac impairment and in the elderly; do not
use in patients with preexisting severe gastrointestinal narrowing; pregnancy risk category C

FIGURE 5.25. Paliperidone is the active metabolite of risperidone (Figure 5.20) and
thus has a similar profile. It is a serotonin 2A/dopamine 2 antagonist and also
blocks alpha 2 adrenergic receptors, which may contribute to efficacy for depression. Receptor "X" in the icon above represents the unclear actions that some atypical antipsychotics have on the insulin system, where they change cellular insulin
resistance and increase fasting plasma triglyceride levels.

Iloperidone

Iloperidone
FANAPT

Dosage Range:
12–24 mg/day in 2 divided doses for schizophrenia

Approved For:
Schizophrenia

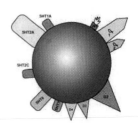

Pearls:
Not studied in PTSD but potent alpha 1 adrenergic blockade suggests potential utility as adjunct for nightmares; must titrate slowly to avoid orthostatic hypotension; weight gain and sedation can be common; do not use in patients taking QTc-prolonging agents or in those with known history of QTc prolongation, recent acute myocardial infarction, or uncompensated heart failure; use with caution in patients with other cardiac impairment and in the elderly; do not use in patients with hepatic impairment; pregnancy risk category C

FIGURE 5.26. In addition to being a serotonin 2A/dopamine 2 antagonist, iloperidone is a potent antagonist at alpha 1 adrenergic receptors, which may contribute to efficacy for treating nightmares. Iloperidone also blocks serotonin 2C, 6, and 7 receptors as well as alpha 2 adrenergic receptors, which could contribute to efficacy for depression.

Asenapine

Asenapine
SAPHRIS

Dosage Range:
10 mg/day in 2 divided doses for schizophrenia;
20 mg/day in 2 divided doses for bipolar mania

Approved For:
Schizophrenia, acute mania/mixed mania

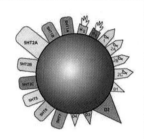

Pearls:
Not studied in PTSD but rationale for use based on shared chemical structure and binding profile with mirtazapine; must be administered sublingually; weight gain is not unusual; sedation can be common; do not use in patients with severe renal impairment; use with caution in patients with cardiac impairment and in the elderly; pregnancy risk category C

FIGURE 5.27. Asenapine has widespread actions on the serotonergic, dopaminergic, and noradrenergic systems and also blocks histamine 1 receptors. The relevance of its actions at many receptors is not yet known, but serotonin 2C and alpha 2 antagonist properties may contribute to antidepressant actions, while histamine 1 antagonism may be largely responsible for its sedative effects.

Anticonvulsants

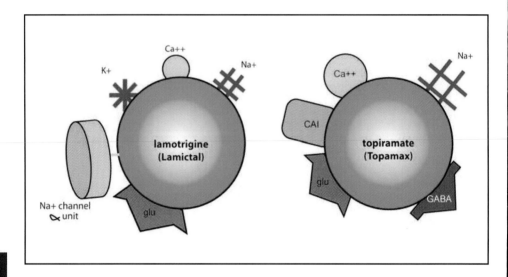

FIGURE 5.28. Many anticonvulsants are used in the treatment of mental illnesses, most frequently in bipolar disorder. They are not well studied in PTSD, though there are small preliminary studies with lamotrigine and topiramate. The mechanisms of action of anticonvulsants are unique and not well understood, but many seem to have effects on the GABA-ergic and glutamatergic systems. Lamotrigine may work by blocking the alpha subunit of voltage-sensitive sodium channels; it may also reduce glutamate release and have actions at other ion channels for calcium and potassium. Topiramate may interfere with voltage-sensitive sodium and/or calcium channels in order to enhance GABA and reduce glutamate actions, and is also a weak inhibitor of carbonic anhydrase.

Lamotrigine and Topiramate

Lamotrigine
Lamictal

Dosage Range:
Bipolar disorder: 100–200 mg/day for monotherapy; 100 mg/day with valproate; 400 mg/day with enzyme-inducing anticonvulsant drugs

Approved For:
Maintenance treatment of bipolar I disorder; partial seizures, ages 2 and older (adjunct); generalized seizures of Lennox-Gastaut syndrome, ages 2 and older (adjunct); conversion to monotherapy in adults with partial seizures who are receiving carbamazepine, phenytoin, phenobarbital, primidone, or valproate

Pearls:
Limited preliminary evidence of efficacy in PTSD; may be useful for patients with comorbid depression; weight gain and sedation are unusual; serious rash can occur; very important to follow dosing guidelines and titration schedule in order to reduce risk of side effects including rash; dose should be halved if used in conjunction with valproate; use lower dose for patients with renal impairment, but may need supplemental doses for patients receiving hemodialysis; use lower dose for patients with hepatic impairment; use with caution in patients with cardiac impairment; pregnancy risk category C

Topiramate
Topamax

Dosage Range:
Bipolar disorder: 50–300 mg/day (adjunct)

Approved For:
Partial onset seizures, ages 2–16 and adults (adjunct); primary generalized tonic-clonic seizures, ages 2–16 and adults (adjunct); seizures associated with Lennox-Gastaut syndrome, ages 2 and older; migraine prophylaxis

Pearls:
Limited preliminary evidence of efficacy in PTSD; may help reduce alcohol intake; can also help pain states associated with PTSD, especially migraine; sedation can be common; weight gain is unusual, some patients may experience weight loss; metabolic acidosis and kidney stones can occur; use lower dose for patients with renal impairment; use with caution in patients with hepatic or cardiac impairment; pregnancy risk category C

FIGURE 5.29. Brief clinical characteristics of some adjunct medications prescribed for PTSD.

Alcohol Dependence/Withdrawal Treatments

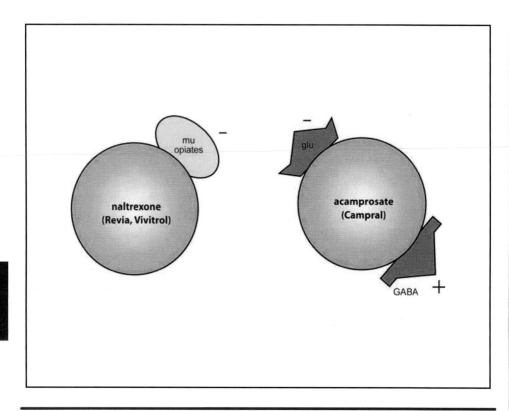

FIGURE 5.30. Alcohol abuse is one of the most common comorbidities in PTSD. Two pharmacologic options for treating alcohol abuse/dependence are naltrexone and acamprosate.

Naltrexone is a mu opioid receptor antagonist that can reduce the pleasurable effects of drinking and thus both decrease heavy drinking and increase abstinence. Adherence is an important consideration, however, and may be enhanced by administering naltrexone as a once monthly intramuscular injection (naltrexone XR).

Acamprosate is a derivative of the amino acid taurine and, like alcohol, both reduces excitatory glutamate neurotransmission and enhances GABA neurotransmission. It is therefore able to "substitute" for alcohol during withdrawal to mitigate the adverse effects and increase the likelihood of abstinence.

Naltrexone and Acamprosate

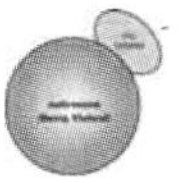

Naltrexone
Revia, Vivitrol

Dosage Range:
Oral 50 mg/day; injection 380 mg/4 weeks

Approved For:
Alcohol dependence; blockade of effects of exogenously administered opioids (oral)

Pearls:
May be preferred if the goal is reduced-risk drinking; weight gain is unusual; sedation is not unusual; can cause hepatocellular injury when given in excessive doses; do not use in patients with acute hepatitis or liver failure; do not use if patient is taking opioid analgesics, is currently dependent on opioids or in acute opiate withdrawal, has failed the naloxone challenge or had a positive urine screen for opioids; pregnancy risk category C

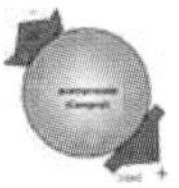

Acamprosate
Campral

Dosage Range:
666 mg three times daily

Approved For:
Maintenance of alcohol abstinence

Pearls:
May be preferred if the goal is complete abstinence; may be less effective in situations in which the patient has not yet abstained; weight gain and sedation are unusual; use lower dose for patients with moderate renal impairment; do not use in patients with severe renal impairment; pregnancy risk category C

FIGURE 5.31. Brief clinical characteristics of some adjunct medications prescribed for alcohol dependence/withdrawal.

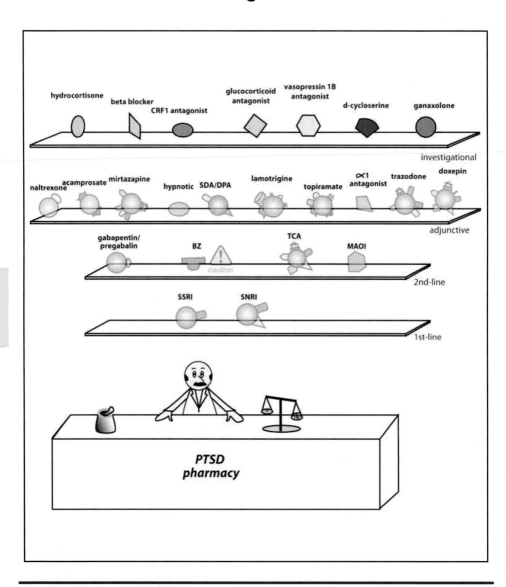

FIGURE 5.32. Several pharmacologic mechanisms are under investigation for their potential use in PTSD.

Can PTSD Be Prevented?
Beta Blockers

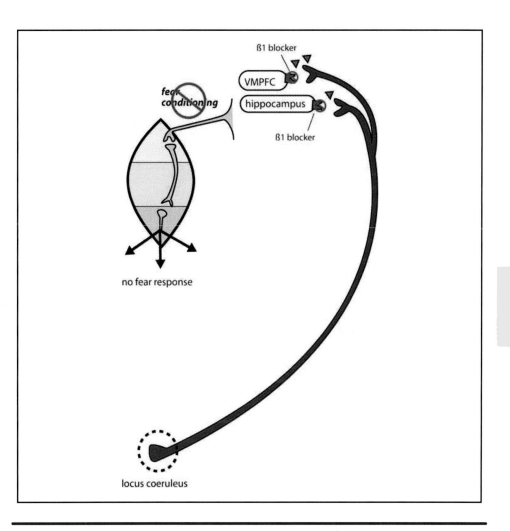

FIGURE 5.33. There is some research to suggest that administration of beta adrenergic blockers immediately following exposure to trauma could block fear conditioning before it even occurs. Specifically, blockade of beta receptors in the ventromedial prefrontal cortex (VMPFC) and hippocampus may prevent input from reaching the amygdala and thus prevent synaptic changes that lead to fear conditioning. Though intriguing, this is not yet a proven treatment strategy.

Can PTSD Be Prevented?
Hydrocortisone

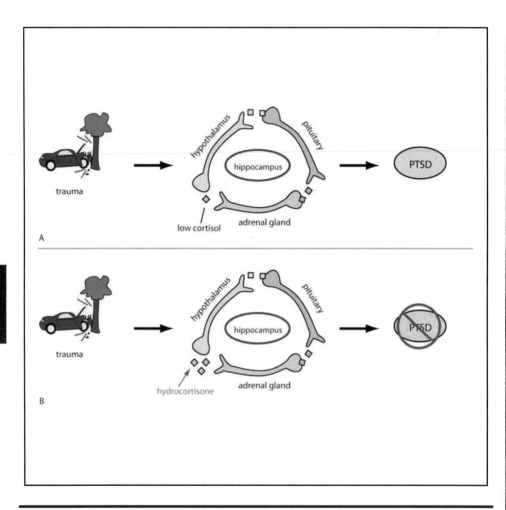

FIGURE 5.34. Another potential preemptive treatment for PTSD is hydrocortisone. Decreased cortisol levels have been demonstrated in PTSD patients (Figure 2.7), and in fact low cortisol levels at the time of exposure to a traumatic event predict development of PTSD (A), so it is reasonable that administering cortisol immediately following exposure could prevent development of the disorder (B). There is some empirical support for this strategy, although as with beta adrenergic blockers it is preliminary.

D-Cycloserine

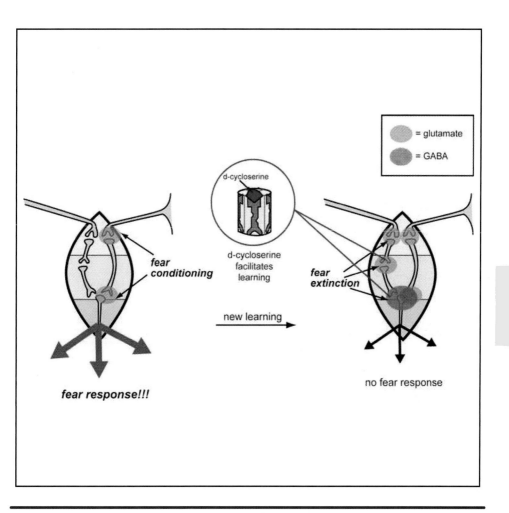

FIGURE 5.35. Fear conditioning (Figure 1.10) is not readily reversed, but it can be suppressed through fear extinction, a type of new learning in which there is a progressive reduction of the response to a feared stimulus when it is repeatedly presented without adverse consequences. Strengthening of synapses involved in fear extinction could help enhance the development of fear extinction learning in the amygdala and reduce symptoms of PTSD. D-cycloserine is an NMDA receptor co-agonist that may contribute to extinction of fear responses during exposure therapy (see Figure 6.2) by increasing the efficiency of glutamate neurotransmission at such synapses.

Potential Targets within the HPA Axis

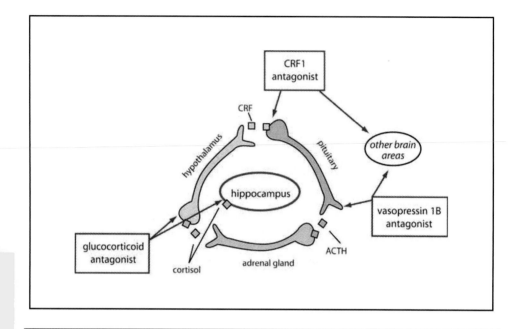

FIGURE 5.36. The central role of the HPA axis in stress responses (Figure 1.6) and in PTSD (Figure 2.7) is well established. There are several potential therapeutic targets within the HPA axis under investigation for PTSD.

One such approach is CRF1 receptor antagonists. CRF is elevated in PTSD; thus blocking its actions may prevent the abnormal stress response and alleviate symptoms. CRF1 receptors are also present in the brain outside the HPA axis, and actions there could theoretically have therapeutic effects as well.

Another approach is glucocorticoid receptor antagonists, which can compete with cortisol at the glucocorticoid receptor and result in lack of expression of glucocorticoid genes, again potentially preventing the abnormal stress response as well as hippocampal atrophy.

A third approach is antagonism of vasopressin 1B receptors. Stimulation of vasopressin 1B receptors contributes to release of ACTH during stress reactions; thus blocking these receptors may prevent complications within the HPA axis. As with CRF1 receptors, vasopressin 1B receptors are present in the brain outside of the HPA axis and activity there could also theoretically be therapeutic.

Neuroactive Steroid:
Ganaxolone

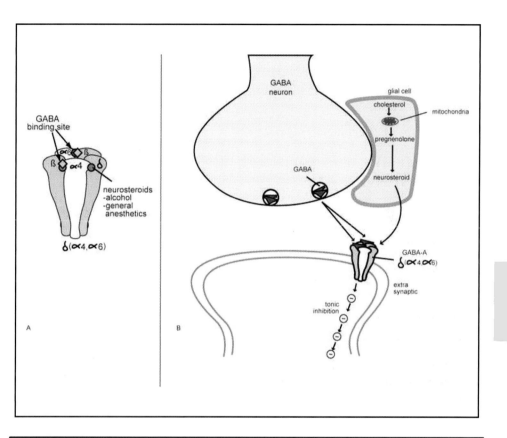

FIGURE 5.37. Neuroactive steroids are another potential novel treatment option for PTSD. Endogenous neuroactive steroids such as allopregnanolone and its equipotent stereoisomer, pregnanolone, bind to the delta subtype of GABA-A receptors (A) to facilitate tonic GABA neurotransmission (B). Because GABA plays a central role in the experience and expression (or suppression) of anxiety (Figure 3.11), it is reasonable that reduced activity of these neurosteroids would be anxiogenic. In fact, some research suggests that there is a block in the synthesis of these two endogenous neuroactive steroids in individuals with PTSD.

Ganaxolone is a synthetic, 3-beta-methylated derivative of allopregnanolone that is currently under development for the treatment of epilepsy. Although it is not yet being studied in PTSD, there is hope that eventually such research will be pursued.

|

Chapter 6

Cognitive Behavioral Therapy (CBT) for PTSD

Cognitive behavioral therapy (CBT) is a structured form of psychotherapy that includes both behavioral modification strategies and cognitive therapies. There are many different types of CBT, all of which are intended to help patients learn new responses to life situations. Most if not all patients with PTSD should have CBT as part of their treatment regimen. In this chapter, the methods for the best-evidenced cognitive and behavioral therapies for patients with PTSD are explained.

Cognitive Behavioral Therapy (CBT):
First-line Options

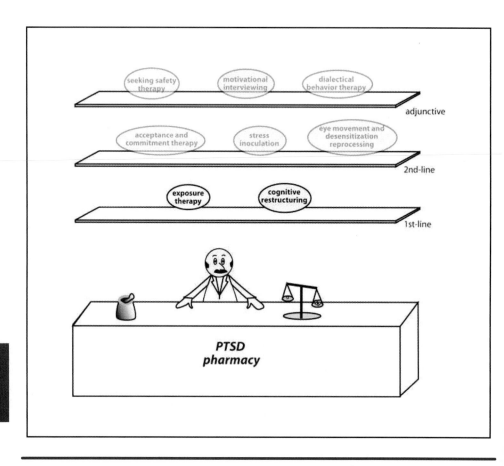

FIGURE 6.1. Cognitive behavioral therapy (CBT) for PTSD is designed to modify the behaviors and thoughts/beliefs that developed in response to trauma. First-line therapies include exposure therapy and cognitive restructuring.

Exposure Therapy

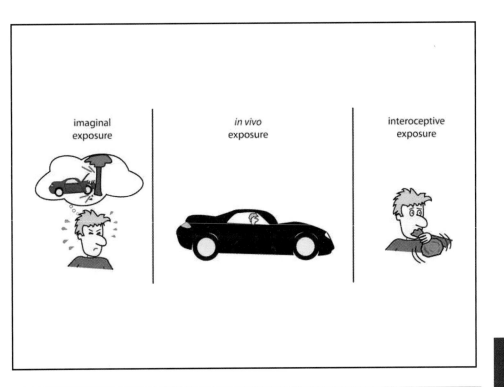

imaginal exposure   *in vivo* exposure   interoceptive exposure

FIGURE 6.2. Exposure therapy for PTSD involves exposing the patient to feared stimuli associated with the traumatic event for repeated and prolonged periods of time. There are several forms of exposure therapy: imaginal, which involves repeatedly recounting traumatic memories; in vivo, which is exposure to feared stimuli in real life; and interoceptive, which involves experiencing feared physical sensations. Combining multiple types of exposure therapy is generally most effective.

Exposure therapy can target reexperiencing symptoms (by reducing fear associated with thinking about the trauma) and avoidance behaviors (by reducing fear associated with confronting trauma-related stimuli that are not actually dangerous), as well as reduce general hyperarousal. In addition, by increasing the patient's perceived control over fear, this can facilitate processing of the traumatic memory (help patients "make sense" of it).

Cognitive Restructuring

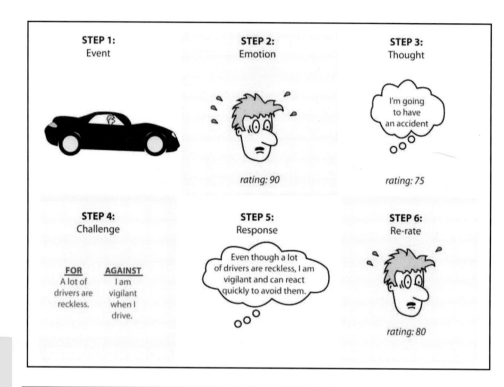

FIGURE 6.3. Cognitive restructuring is a process by which patients learn to evaluate and modify inaccurate and unhelpful thoughts (e.g., "It was my fault I was raped"). Adjusting how one thinks about a traumatic event can presumably alter one's emotional response to it, and in fact cognitive restructuring particularly seems to help address emotions such as shame and guilt. It can be used alone but is often used as an adjunct to exposure therapy.

There are six main steps of cognitive restructuring: (1) identify a distressing event/thought; (2) identify and rate (0–100) emotions related to the event/thought; (3) identify automatic thoughts associated with the emotions, rate the degree to which one believes them, and select one to challenge; (4) identify evidence in support of and against the thought; (5) generate a response to the thought using the evidence for/against (even though <evidence for>, in fact <evidence against>) and rate the degree of belief in the response; (6) rerate emotion related to the event/thought.

Cognitive Behavioral Therapy (CBT):
Second-line Options

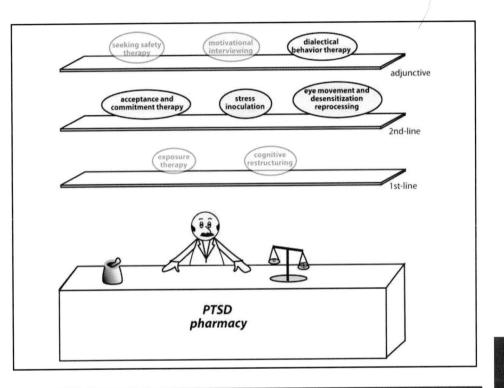

FIGURE 6.4. Second-line CBT options include stress inoculation training (SIT) and eye movement desensitization and reprocessing therapy (EMDR). Two additional strategies include dialectical behavior therapy (DBT), which may be useful as an adjunct, and acceptance and commitment therapy (ACT).

Stress Inoculation Training

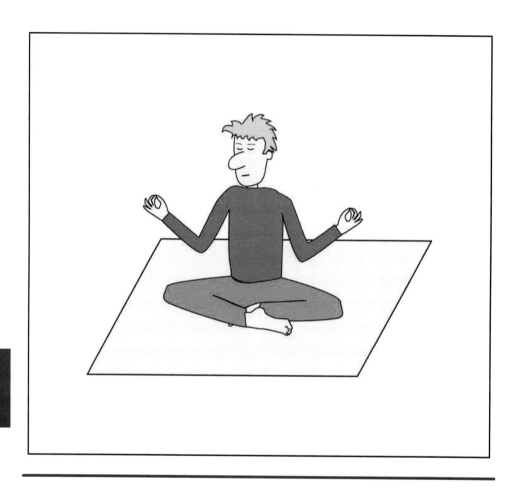

FIGURE 6.5. There are other therapies that may be considered second-line. Stress inoculation training (SIT) is an anxiety management approach in which patients learn techniques such as relaxation, assertive communication skills, thought stopping (distracting oneself from distressing thoughts), and guided self-dialogue (replacing irrational negative internal dialogue with rational thoughts).

Eye Movement Desensitization and Reprocessing

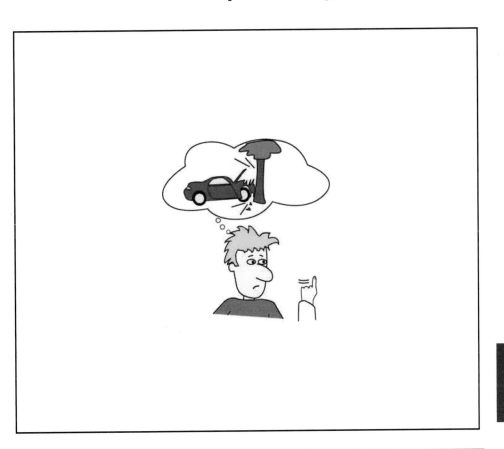

FIGURE 6.6. Another second-line strategy, eye movement desensitization and re-processing (EMDR), is a technique in which patients recount traumatic experiences while focusing on a moving object (e.g., the therapist's finger), with the intention that this facilitates the processing of the traumatic memory. There is empirical support for this approach, though not as much as for exposure therapy and cognitive restructuring.

Dialectical Behavior Therapy

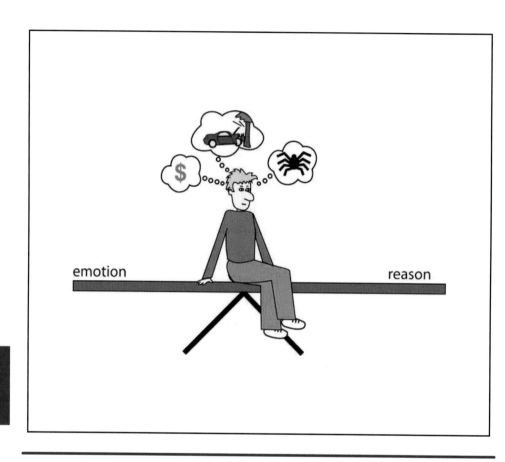

FIGURE 6.7. Dialectical behavior therapy (DBT) is designed to address destructive behaviors and emotion regulation in borderline personality disorder, but has been used in other disorders including PTSD. DBT stresses validation, balance between acceptance and change, and mindfulness (being present with the moment and aware of both your emotions and your thoughts). Because DBT teaches patients to be aware in the moment and accept unpleasant emotions, it may be particularly useful as an adjunct for patients who dissociate during exposure therapy.

Acceptance and Commitment Therapy

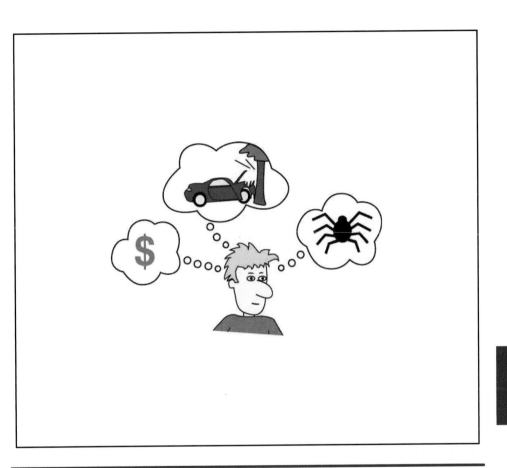

FIGURE 6.8. A similar therapy, acceptance and commitment therapy (ACT), involves acceptance of thoughts and anxiety as experiences that a person can have while still living a life in accordance with one's values.

Cognitive Behavioral Therapy (CBT):
Adjunct Options

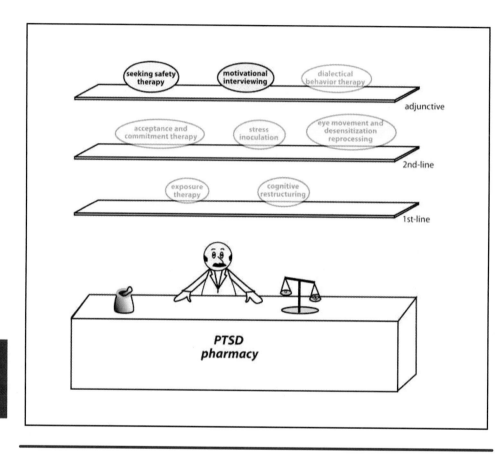

FIGURE 6.9. Seeking safety therapy and motivational interviewing may be used for patients with comorbid substance dependence/abuse.

Seeking Safety Therapy

Interpersonal Topics
Asking for Help
Honesty
Setting Boundaries in Relationships
Healthy Relationships
Community Resources
Healing from Anger
Getting Others to Support Your Recovery

Behavioral Topics
Detaching from Emotional Pain: Grounding
Taking Good Care of Yourself
Red and Green Flags
Commitment
Coping with Triggers
Respecting Your Time
Self-nurturing

Cognitive Topics
PTSD: Taking Back Your Power
Compassion
When Substances Control You
Recovery Thinking
Integrating the Split Self
Creating Meaning
Discovery

Combination Topics
Introduction to Treatment /
Case Management
Safety
The Life Choices Game (Review)
Termination

FIGURE 6.10. Seeking safety therapy is a technique specifically developed for individuals with substance abuse and trauma histories. It is an integrated treatment approach in which both PTSD and substance abuse are addressed simultaneously, with the main goal being to help patients attain safety in their lives (in terms of relationships, thought processes, behaviors, and emotions). Seeking safety offers 25 treatment topics based on four content areas: cognitive, behavioral, interpersonal, and case management. The treatment can be customized for each individual patient, using whatever combination of treatment topics that best suits the patient's needs. A clinician guide and client handouts are available for each treatment topic.

Motivational Interviewing

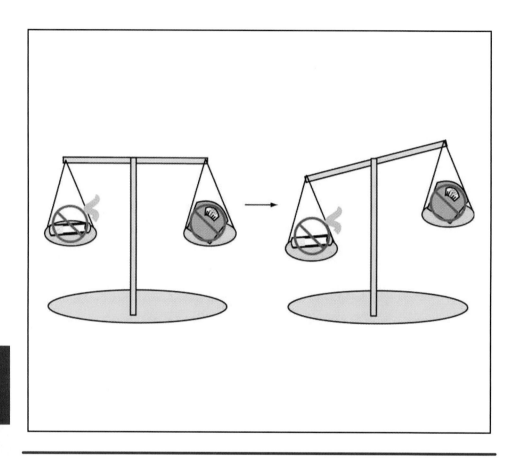

FIGURE 6.11. Motivational interviewing is patient-focused counseling with the direct goal of enhancing one's motivation to change by helping explore and resolve ambivalence (e.g., "I want to stop smoking, but I'm afraid I'll gain weight"). It was originally developed to help individuals with problem drinking but can be used in the treatment of patients with other forms of substance abuse and dependence. With motivational interviewing the clinician is a facilitator, helping the patient identify, articulate, and resolve his or her own ambivalence without direct persuasion, confrontation, or coercion.

Caring for Patients With PTSD

Treatment of PTSD includes both nonpharmacological and pharmacological options, with many patients likely benefiting from a combination of the two. PTSD can be a very difficult disorder to treat, and outcomes in general may not be as positive as those for other anxiety disorders or for depression, particularly with respect to pharmacological treatments. Most patients with PTSD also have at least one comorbid disorder, further complicating the clinical picture.

This chapter reviews diagnostic and treatment strategies for patients with PTSD, including consideration of comorbidities. Prior to beginning any treatment for PTSD, it is important to fully inform the patient about the disorder and its treatments, including realistic expectations of treatment outcomes.

Screening and Assessment

ASSESSMENT TOOLS	NOTES
Primary Care Posttraumatic Stress Disorder Screen (PC-PTSD)	4-item self-administered tool; yes–no measure; each item assesses one dimension of PTSD (reexperiencing, avoidance, numbing, hyper-arousal); 2 or more yes answers warrants further evaluation Used by military branches
Posttraumatic Stress Disorder Checklist (PCL)	19-item self-administered tool; 0–4 point scale; based on DSM-IV criteria; civilian and military versions; recommended cutoff score of 50, though some suggest it could be lower Used by military branches
Posttraumatic Diagnostic Scale (PDS)	4-part self-administered tool; parts 1 and 2 assess trauma history while parts 3 and 4 assess for PTSD symptoms and functional impairment, respectively; part 3 uses a 0–3 point scale, is based on DSM-IV criteria, and has a cutoff score of 15
Davidson Trauma Scale (DTS)	17-item self-administered tool; both frequency and severity are rated for each item; 0–4 point scale; based on DSM-IV criteria; cutoff score of 40
SPAN	4-item self-administered tool; derived from Davidson Trauma Scale; cutoff score of 5 or more
Trauma Questionnaire (TQ), Stressful Life Events Screening Questionnaire (SLESQ)	Evaluate for presence of traumatic event

TABLE 7.1. This table gives an overview of screening and assessment tools available to clinicians for PTSD. The tools included here are self-administered, have documented validity, and are relatively easy to implement in clinical practice. The most commonly used clinician-rated scale in multicenter medication trials is the Clinician-Administered PTSD Scale, part 2 (CAPS-2, not shown).

Screening for Suicidality

Psychiatric illnesses	Comorbid affective disorders, substance abuse, Cluster B personality disorders, etc.
History	Prior suicide attempts, aborted attempts or self harm; medical diagnoses, family history of suicide / attempts / mental illness
Individual strengths / vulnerabilities	Coping skills; personality traits; past responses to stress; capacity for reality testing; tolerance of psychological pain
Psychosocial situation	Acute and chronic stressors; changes in status; quality of support; religious beliefs
Suicidality	Past and present suicidal ideation, plans, behaviors, intent; methods
Warning signs	Emotions (serious depression; acute agitation, anxiety, insomnia; feeling overwhelmed or that there is no way out) Behaviors (withdrawal from friends and activities, increase in substance use, impulsiveness, putting self in danger, giving away possessions, finalizing personal affairs, any unusual behavior) Expressions (death themes in letters, notes; talking or hinting about suicide; stating a desire to die)

TABLE 7.2. This table summarizes factors to evaluate when screening patients for suicide risk. Suicide assessment should not be rushed and should be repeatedly periodically. It is not uncommon for patients to be untruthful when responding to questions about suicidal ideation and intent; thus responses should not merely be taken at face value. Instead, the other factors listed here as well as intuition should be used when making clinical decisions.

Assessing for Comorbid Disorders and Complications

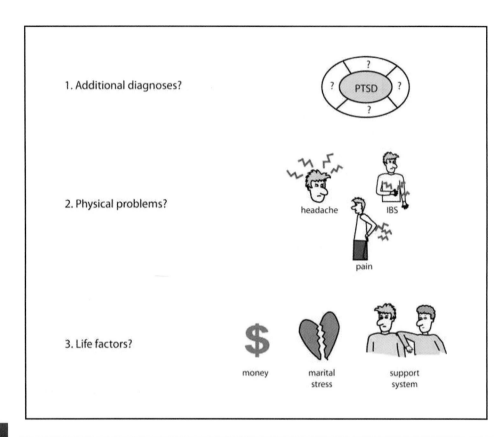

FIGURE 7.1. Because of the high rates of comorbid disorders in patients with PTSD, which can affect the selection and sequence of treatment, it is important to assess for such disorders prior to determining a treatment plan. Physical illnesses may also affect clinical decisions and should be evaluated; common problems in patients with PTSD include headaches, irritable bowel syndrome, and chronic pain. In addition, it is important to assess for life factors that may either help or hinder treatment, such as abusive relationships, marital discord, financial difficulties, life demands, and support systems.

Cognitive Behavioral Therapy (CBT)

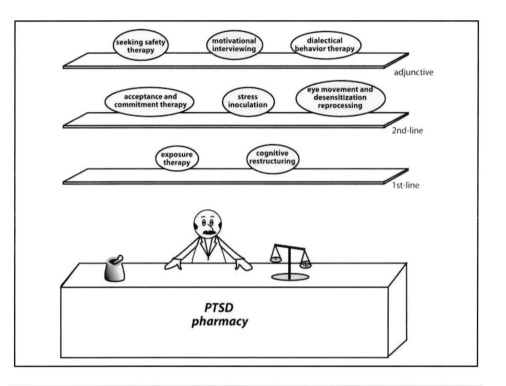

FIGURE 7.2. Shown here is a summary of the first-line, second-line, and adjunctive cognitive behavioral therapy (CBT) and psychotherapy options described in Chapter 6. CBT should typically be included in the management of any patient with PTSD, but the particular therapy used will vary depending on the particular patient and requires consideration of comorbid disorders, life factors, and the patient's readiness to accept treatment.

Pharmacological Treatments

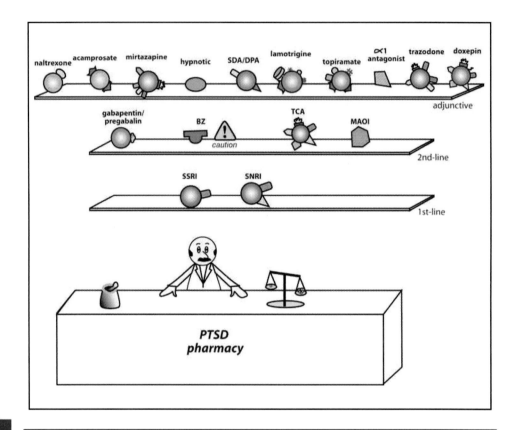

FIGURE 7.3. Shown here is a summary of the first-line, second-line, and adjunctive medication options for PTSD. First-line medications include the selective serotonin reuptake inhibitors and serotonin norepinephrine reuptake inhibitors, with only paroxetine and sertraline approved by the Food and Drug Administration (FDA) for this indication. There is limited evidence for any other medications as monotherapy for PTSD, and in fact even first-line treatments often leave patients with residual symptoms. SSRIs and SNRIs were covered in detail in Chapter 4, while second-line, adjunct, and investigational options were covered in Chapter 5.

Treating PTSD and Comorbid Substance Use/Abuse

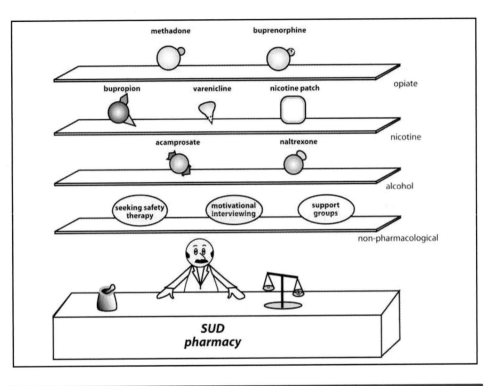

FIGURE 7.4. The approach to treatment for patients with comorbid PTSD and substance dependence/abuse may vary depending on the degree of dependence or addiction. Patients with significant problems with substance dependence/abuse may need to address that first before beginning PTSD treatment, particularly cognitive behavioral therapy. Other patients may be able to address both simultaneously or begin treatment for PTSD first. For patients with nicotine dependence it may be best to address PTSD symptoms prior to attempting smoking cessation. In all cases, substance use should be carefully monitored during treatment, and any increase in substance use should be managed promptly.

Specific pharmacologic treatments for substance dependence/abuse that may be used as adjuncts to PTSD treatment include naltrexone and acamprosate for alcohol use, methadone and buprenorphine for opiate dependence, and bupropion, varenicline, and nicotine replacement for nicotine dependence. Non-pharmacological strategies include seeking safety therapy, motivational interviewing, and support groups.

Treating PTSD and Comorbid Depression

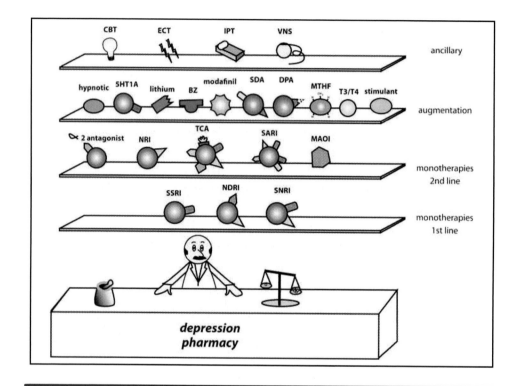

FIGURE 7.5. In general, first-line pharmacological treatments for depression are the same as those for anxiety disorders, with first-line options generally being selective serotonin reuptake inhibitors (SSRI) and serotonin norepinephrine reuptake inhibitors (SNRI). Bupropion, a norepinephrine and dopamine reuptake inhibitor (NDRI), is a first-line option for depression as well and may particularly help patients with fatigue and cognitive symptoms. In addition, there are many other second-line, adjunct, and ancillary treatment options for depression, many of which overlap with those for PTSD. In general there is a larger body of evidence for effectiveness of pharmacological treatments in depression than there is in PTSD.

Cognitive behavioral therapy (CBT) can also be an important part of depression treatment. Combining pharmacological and cognitive behavioral therapy may be particularly important for patients with comorbid depression and PTSD in order to reach a positive outcome.

Treating PTSD and Comorbid Anxiety Disorders

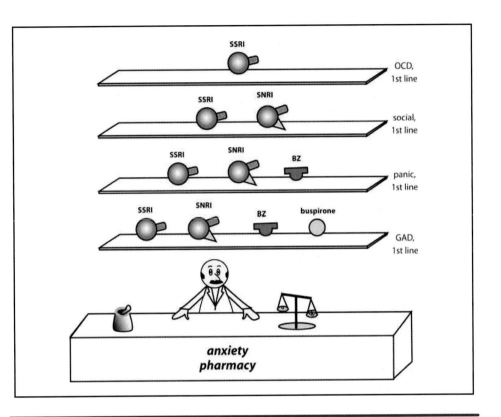

FIGURE 7.6. There is quite a bit of overlap between both the pharmacological and non-pharmacological treatment options for PTSD and other anxiety disorders, and in many cases symptoms of comorbid anxiety disorders will improve with PTSD treatment, particularly if symptoms of the comorbid disorder are functionally related to PTSD. If the disorders are truly distinct, however, then cognitive behavioral techniques will likely need to be targeted to each disorder. Cognitive behavioral therapies can either be simultaneous or sequential, depending on the needs of the patient.

With respect to pharmacological options, the main difference between treatment for PTSD and other anxiety disorders is that benzodiazepines have well established efficacy in generalized anxiety disorder and panic disorder, whereas there is a lack of evidence for their use in PTSD. However, they should still be used with caution in patients with PTSD and comorbid anxiety.

Treating PTSD and Comorbid Sleep Problems

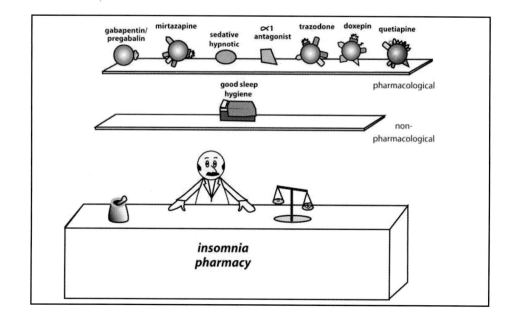

FIGURE 7.7. Most patients with PTSD have problems with insomnia, typically manifested as difficulty initiating or maintaining sleep. For some patients sleep difficulties can resolve with PTSD treatment, but it is not uncommon for insomnia to remain a problem even after other symptoms have resolved. For these patients it may be necessary to address insomnia directly.

When selecting treatment for insomnia, it is important to determine both the underlying cause, if possible, as well as contributing factors. For example, many patients with PTSD will feel a sense of heightened danger at night; furthermore, depending on the particular trauma history, the bedroom itself may be considered a dangerous environment. These patients may therefore keep the light on or have television or music playing for comfort, all of which are contrary to good sleep hygiene. Thus, in addition to addressing fears associated with sleeping, patients should be educated on proper sleep hygiene.

If insomnia persists, medication may be necessary. There are many pharmacologic options available, including sedating antidepressants, quetiapine, and sedative hypnotics. Alpha 1 antagonists may help reduce nightmares, while alpha 2 delta ligands can improve slow-wave sleep.

Treating PTSD and Comorbid Chronic Pain

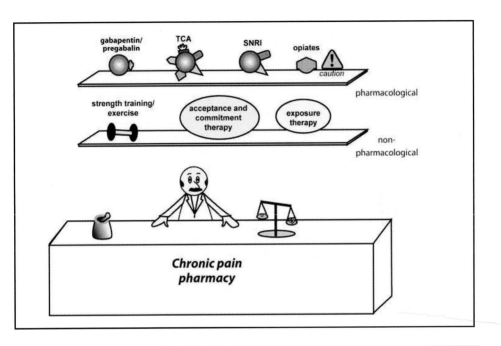

FIGURE 7.8. There is limited research on the treatment of comorbid PTSD and chronic pain. When determining a treatment plan for chronic pain it is important to assess not only pain severity, location, distribution, and triggers, but also attitudes and beliefs about pain, existing coping methods, and functional impairments.

Several cognitive behavioral therapies that are used for PTSD can also be applied to the treatment of chronic pain, including exposure therapy (both in vivo exposure to pain-related activities and interoceptive exposure to feared physical sensations) and acceptance and commitment therapy. Exercise can also be beneficial for reducing chronic pain and may be therapeutic for arousal symptoms as well.

Multiple pharmacologic options for PTSD are also treatments for chronic pain. These include the first-line serotonin norepinephrine reuptake inhibitors (SNRIs), tricyclic antidepressants (TCAs), and gabapentin and pregabalin. Other antidepressants and anticonvulsants are also often used to treat chronic pain. Opiates are frequently prescribed, but such use should be cautious due to the risk of dependence and addiction; this may be a particular concern for PTSD patients, who already have heightened risk for substance abuse and dependence.

| Chapter 8

Unique Considerations
for the Military Population

By virtue of their occupation, individuals in the military are at heightened risk for exposure to traumatic events. This has become particularly apparent in recent years, as the wars in Afghanistan and Iraq have contributed to drastic increases in the rates of PTSD, depression, and suicide among service members. There has also been a rise in the rates of traumatic brain injuries (TBI), as advances in protective equipment have increased the chances of survival from injuries that previously would have been fatal. This chapter focuses on risks and complicating factors that are particularly relevant to the military population, with emphasis on the relationship between PTSD and the potential long-term effects of mild TBI.

Military Personnel:
A Population at Risk

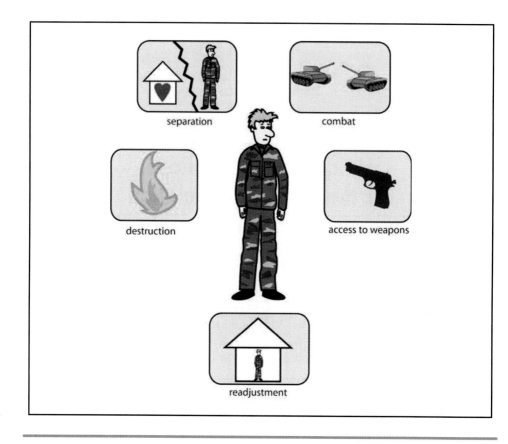

FIGURE 8.1. The experience of combat can involve having one's own life threatened, observing death or injury of others, being unable to protect others from harm, or being the agent of killing or harm to others. In addition, deployed troops witness the often devastating effects of war on civilians and their communities.

The high rates of exposure to trauma combined with the separation from loved ones during deployment, and the difficulty of readjusting to life following deployment (particularly for reserves), create a uniquely elevated risk of PTSD for service members. Alcohol and drug abuse are also common in the military population and can complicate the presentation of PTSD as well as increase risk for suicidal behavior. The ready access to weapons and training in how to use them are additional concerns for individuals with suicidal ideation, plans, or intent.

Impact of the Iraq and Afghanistan Wars

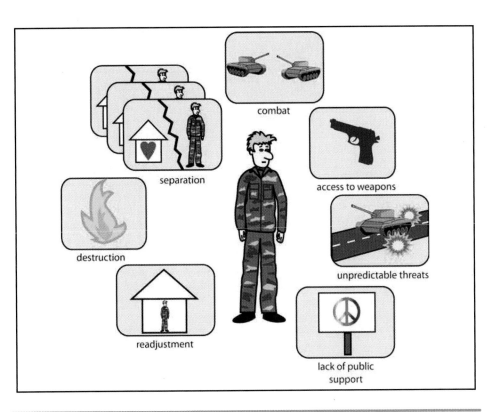

FIGURE 8.2. Recognition of these unique considerations for the military population is particularly important in light of the wars in Iraq and Afghanistan, which have contributed to drastic rises in the rates of mental illnesses in the military, most notably PTSD and depression, as well as unprecedented numbers of completed suicides. In fact, as many as a fifth of services members returning from Iraq may have a mental health problem; this may increase to one in four for those who have deployed three or more times. One factor that may make service members in these wars more vulnerable is that the dangers they face on a daily basis are unexpected and unpredictable: instead of a front line, they have improvised explosive devices and roadside bombs. Prolonged and frequent deployments are also common and can compound the effects of separation from family and difficulties with reintegration as well as potentially increase the likelihood of exposure to combat (see Figure 8.3). Relative lack of public support for the wars in Iraq and Afghanistan can negatively impact troop morale and may be an important modifying factor as well.

More Combat Exposure Increases Risk of PTSD

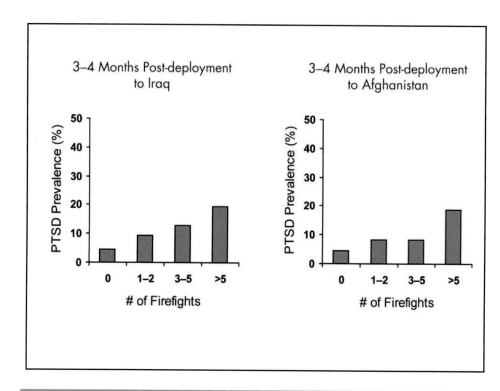

FIGURE 8.3. Risk for development of PTSD may increase with greater exposure to combat (e.g., being shot at, knowing someone who was killed, killing another individual). In fact, a linear relationship between number of firefights and PTSD prevalence has been shown among soldiers and Marines deployed either to Iraq or to Afghanistan.

Barriers to Care:
Ongoing Stigma and Limited Resources

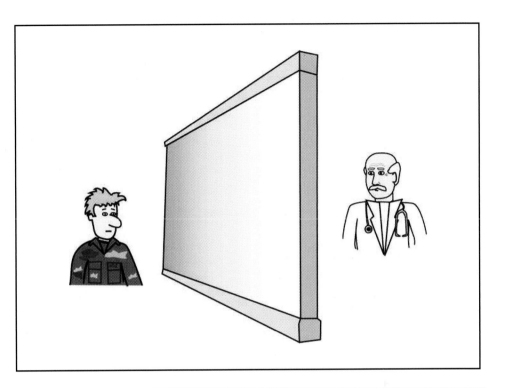

FIGURE 8.4. A core concern with respect to service members exposed to trauma is the ongoing stigma associated with mental illness and with individuals who receive such diagnoses. Despite destigmatization and education programs on mental illness that have been implemented in the various branches of the military, there may still be a significant proportion of service members who doubt that PTSD is a real illness that can result from military service. This stigma and lack of support for individuals with trauma-related mental illness can significantly limit and/or undermine the quality of care that they receive, if they are even willing to seek care at all.

Further complicating the diagnosis and treatment of service members with mental illnesses is the fact that there is a major shortage of mental health staffing within the army. Other medical professionals within the army do not have extensive mental health training; thus access to qualified mental health professionals is a considerable problem.

Physical Symptoms as a Common Presentation of PTSD in Veterans

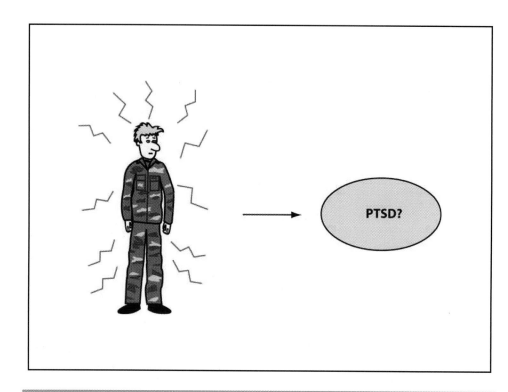

FIGURE 8.5. Service members with PTSD may be likely to present with a number of physical symptoms. Physical symptoms including chronic pain can be a common comorbidity to PTSD following injury (Figure 2.10), but may also be associated with PTSD even in the absence of injury. Studies of veterans of the Gulf war and of the Iraq war demonstrate that PTSD is independently associated with diminished general health and greater number of physical symptoms such as abdominal, muscle, joint, and head pain. In fact, among combat veterans seeking treatment for PTSD, as many as two-thirds have a preexisting chronic pain diagnosis. In particular, temporomandibular joint disorders (TMJ) and chronic widespread pain are commonly comorbid with PTSD. It is therefore important to evaluate for PTSD in service members and veterans presenting with physical complaints.

Mild Traumatic Brain Injury (TBI)

Points	Eye Opening Response	Verbal Response	Motor Response
6			Obeys commands for movement
5		Oriented	Purposeful movement to painful stimulus
4	Spontaneous—open with blinking at baseline	Confused conversation, but able to answer questions	Withdraws in response to pain
3	To verbal stimuli, command, speech	Inappropriate words	Flexion in response to pain (decorticate posturing)
2	To pain only (not applied to face)	Incomprehensible speech	Extension response in response to pain (decerebrate posturing)
1	No response	No response	No response

TABLE 8.1. An additional complication for both the differential diagnosis and treatment of PTSD is the high rate of traumatic brain injury (TBI) among service members involved in the Iraq and Afghanistan wars. TBI is defined as a physical or mechanical brain injury causing temporary or permanent impairment of brain function. It can be either open (foreign object penetrating the brain) or closed (blunt force, acceleration/deceleration). Mild TBI is generally defined as an alteration in level of consciousness or a loss of consciousness that lasts up to 30 minutes, with normal computerized tomography (CT) and/or magnetic resonance imaging (MRI) scans and a Glasgow Coma Scale (GCS) score of 13–15 (see above). TBIs are the most frequent physical injury among personnel serving in the current wars, and are typically closed, resulting from explosion or blast injury.

Mild TBI and PTSD:
Can They Co-occur?

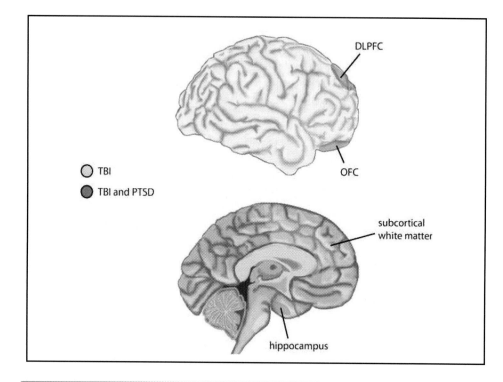

TBI
TBI and PTSD

DLPFC
OFC
subcortical white matter
hippocampus

FIGURE 8.6. There has been controversy over whether it is possible for both PTSD and TBI to result from the same trauma, in large part because TBI generally involves amnesia of the traumatic injury, while PTSD presumably requires recollection of the traumatic event. Examination of large-scale populations has led to the general acceptance that they can co-occur, with divergence in comorbidity rates related to the severity of the TBI. Specifically, severe TBI may actually be protective against PTSD, whereas mild TBI may increase risk, perhaps because resulting cognitive deficits impair the ability to process emotional information related to the trauma.

That both PTSD and TBI could result from the same trauma is not surprising when one considers that the brain regions most vulnerable to TBI are also those associated with symptoms of PTSD (areas shaded in green).

Mild TBI and Persistent Postconcussive Syndrome (PPCS)

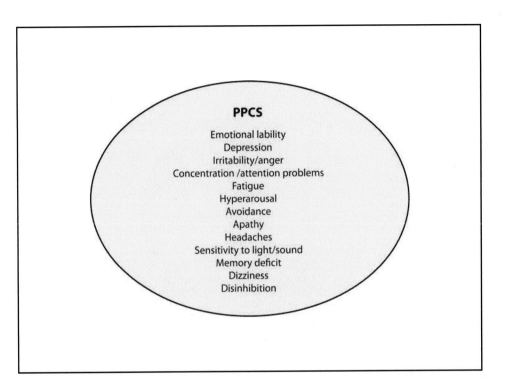

PPCS

Emotional lability
Depression
Irritability/anger
Concentration /attention problems
Fatigue
Hyperarousal
Avoidance
Apathy
Headaches
Sensitivity to light/sound
Memory deficit
Dizziness
Disinhibition

FIGURE 8.7. The majority of individuals who suffer a mild TBI experience acute disorientation, confusion, agitation, and anterograde and retrograde amnesia. Fatigue, headaches, dizziness, sleep disturbances, seizures, and irritability/anger may also occur and often resolve over several days to weeks. A significant minority, however, may experience persistent symptoms that can include the above as well as additional cognitive impairments (memory, attention, concentration, and executive function) and emotional symptoms (apathy, emotional lability, and disinhibition). This constellation of symptoms is termed persistent postconcussive syndrome (PPCS).

PPCS Symptoms:
Are They Really Postconcussive?

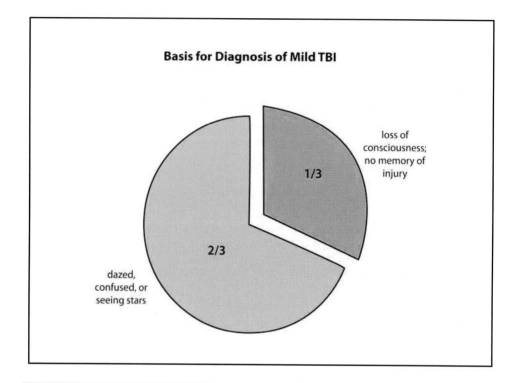

Basis for Diagnosis of Mild TBI

1/3 — loss of consciousness; no memory of injury

2/3 — dazed, confused, or seeing stars

FIGURE 8.8. Although ideally TBI would be diagnosed immediately following injury or blast exposure and using the Glasgow Coma Scale (see Table 8.1), in reality, at least for veterans of Iraq and Afghanistan, the diagnosis is often done retrospectively, months after an injury or exposure to a blast. Further, the diagnosis is typically based on a single positive response to one of three screening questions: (1) did you lose consciousness? (2) were you dazed, confused, or seeing stars? or (3) do you not remember the injury? The problem with this method is that TBI is not the only possible cause of these things—in particular, feeling dazed or confused during a traumatic event may simply be dissociation due to acute stress. Yet almost two-thirds of reported cases of mild TBI among Iraq and Afghanistan war veterans have been identified based on a positive response to that question. Thus many individuals diagnosed with persistent postconcussive syndrome may never have had concussion to begin with.

PPCS and PTSD:
Symptom Overlap

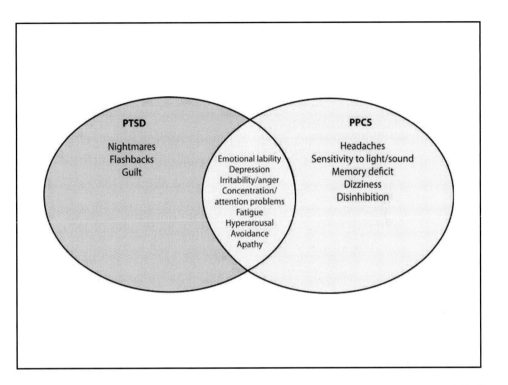

FIGURE 8.9. In fact, many individuals diagnosed with persistent postconcussive syndrome (PPCS) may actually have PTSD. There is a great deal of overlap between symptoms of PPCS and those of PTSD (and of other illnesses as well), making it difficult to determine the underlying cause even in individuals with well-documented history of TBI. The shared symptomatology between PTSD and persistent symptoms of TBI may be explained by the overlap in implicated brain regions shown in Figure 8.6.

PPCS or PTSD?

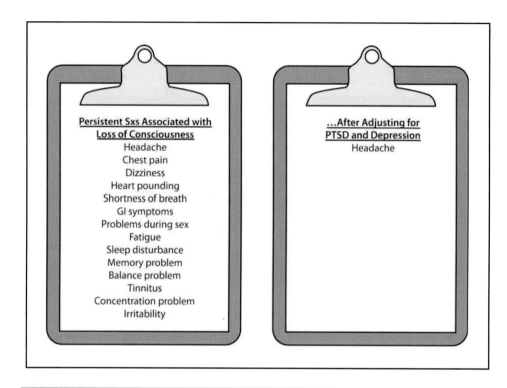

Persistent Sxs Associated with Loss of Consciousness
Headache
Chest pain
Dizziness
Heart pounding
Shortness of breath
GI symptoms
Problems during sex
Fatigue
Sleep disturbance
Memory problem
Balance problem
Tinnitus
Concentration problem
Irritability

...After Adjusting for PTSD and Depression
Headache

FIGURE 8.10. When one considers both the symptom overlap and the fact that most cases of mild TBI in service members are not well-substantiated, it seems likely that there is a large overestimate of the number of individuals with ongoing complications related to brain injury (and a corresponding underestimate of individuals with PTSD). In an analysis of service members reporting mild TBI compared to those with no injury, only persistent headache was associated with loss of consciousness after accounting for PTSD and depression, and no physical health outcomes were associated with altered mental status (dazed/confused or no memory of injury).

Although this section has focused on the military population, it should be noted that TBI does, of course, occur in the civilian population as well. Interestingly, only 3–5% of civilians with mild TBI experience PPCS. In the military population, the estimate based on the current screening process is ten times that.

Treating PTSD in Patients Who Have Had TBI

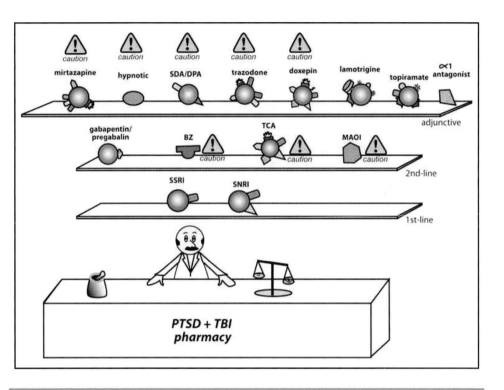

FIGURE 8.11. General treatment recommendations for PTSD in patients who have experienced a TBI are the same as those for PTSD alone; this is true for both pharmacological and non-pharmacological treatments. One should be aware, however, that patients with TBI may be more sensitive to the effects of medications (both therapeutic and side effects) as well as to any potential drug interactions. For patients with co-morbid PTSD and TBI it is best to avoid medications with anticholinergic and sedative effects as well as those that can lower the seizure threshold. Antipsychotics and benzodiazepines in particular are not generally recommended in patients with TBI.

Due to increased sensitivity to medication effects, it is recommended to start at low doses, titrate slowly, monitor vigilantly, and use as few medications as possible. Adherence may be a particular concern for this population: cognitive symptoms may affect one's ability to remember the medication schedule, while impaired concentration, low frustration tolerance, and physical symptoms may impede participation in cognitive behavioral therapy.

Treating PPCS in Patients with PTSD

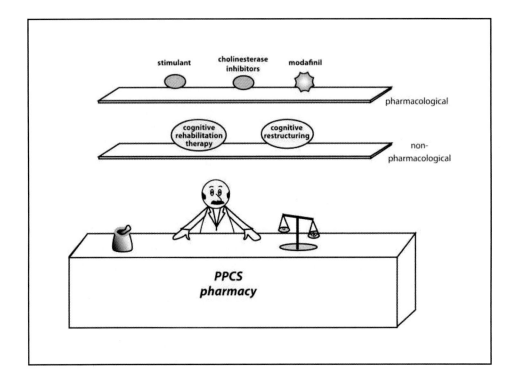

FIGURE 8.12. Individual with postconcussive symptoms may require treatment for impaired cognitive functioning. Cognitive rehabilitation therapy can be used to address problems with attention, memory, and functional communication. Cognitive restructuring may be beneficial for patients who incorrectly attribute symptoms or normal sensations to the brain injury.

Pharmacological treatments for cognition may be used, although this is not well studied in patients with history of TBI and should be done cautiously. Examples of cognitive enhancers include stimulants, cholinesterase inhibitors, and modafinil. Because of the abuse potential of stimulants, these should be used cautiously in patients with PTSD.

Summary

- Anxiety and fear are normal responses to stressors

- The emotional, behavioral, and physical manifestations of anxiety and fear are mediated in large part by amygdala-centered circuits

- Pathological anxiety may develop when repeated stressors and genetic vulnerabilities combine and lead to stress-sensitization within those circuits

- Posttraumatic stress disorder (PTSD) is a particularly prevalent disorder with significant functional consequences

- First-line treatment options for PTSD include cognitive behavioral therapy (CBT—exposure, cognitive restructuring), selective serotonin reuptake inhibitors, and serotonin norepinephrine reuptake inhibitors

- There are also many second-line and adjunct treatment options (pharmacological and non-pharmacological)

- Most patients with PTSD have at least one comorbid disorder, which can affect treatment decisions

- Military personnel face unique circumstances that put them at particular risk for PTSD

5HT	serotonin
ACC	anterior cingulate cortex
ACT	acceptance and commitment therapy
ACTH	adrenocorticotrophin hormone
AMPA	alpha-amino-3-hydroxy-5-methyl-4-isoxazolepropionic acid
BDNF	brain-derived neurotrophic factor
CBT	cognitive behavioral therapy
COMT	catechol-O-methyl-transferase
CR	controlled-release
CRF	corticotrophin releasing factor
CSTC	cortico-striatal-thalamic-cortical
CT	computerized tomography
DA	dopamine
DBT	dialectical behavioral therapy
DLPFC	dorsolateral prefrontal cortex
DRI	dopamine reuptake inhibition
DSM	Diagnostic and Statistical Manual of Mental Disorders
EAAT	excitatory amino acid transporter
EMDR	eye movement desensitization and reprocessing
FDA	Food and Drug Administration
GABA	gamma-aminobutyric acid
GABA-T	gamma-aminobutyric transaminase
GAT	gamma-aminobutyric transporter
GCS	Glasgow Coma Scale
HPA	hypothalamic pituitary adrenal
IR	immediate-release
MAO	monoamine oxidase
MAOI	monoamine oxidase inhibitor
mGluR	metabotropic glutamate receptor
MRI	magnetic resonance imaging
NaSSA	noradrenergic and specific serotonergic antidepressant
NDRI	norepinephrine and dopamine reuptake inhibitor
NE	norepinephrine
NET	norepinephrine transporter

```
NMDA ......... N-methyl-D-aspartate
NOS ........... nitric oxide synthetase
NRI ............. norepinephrine reuptake inhibition
OFC ............. orbitofrontal cortex
PAG ............ periaqueductal grey
PBN ............ parabrachial nucleus
PFC ............. prefrontal cortex
PPCS ........... persistent postconcussive syndrome
PTSD ........... posttraumatic stress disorder
RIMA ........... reversible inhibitor of monoamine oxidase
SERT ........... serotonin transporter
SIT .............. stress inoculation therapy
SNRI ........... serotonin norepinephrine reuptake inhibitor
SRI ............. serotonin reuptake inhibition
SSRI ........... selective serotonin reuptake inhibitor
TBI ............. traumatic brain injury
TCA ............ tricyclic antidepressant
VMPFC ........ ventromedial prefrontal cortex
VSCC .......... voltage-sensitive calcium channel
VSSC .......... voltage-sensitive sodium channel
XR .............. extended-release
```

Suggested Readings*

American Psychiatric Association. Diagnostic and Statistical Manual of Mental Disorders, fourth edition, text revision. Washington, DC: American Psychiatric Association; 2000.

Anderson KC, Insel TR. The promise of extinction research for the prevention and treatment of anxiety disorders. Biol Psychiatry 2006;60:319–21.

Arzt E, Holsboer F. CRF signaling: molecular specificity for drug targeting in the CNS. Trends Pharmacol Sci 2006;27:531–8.

Asmundson GJ, Katz J. Understanding the co-occurrence of anxiety disorders and chronic pain: state-of-the-art. Depress Anx 2009;26:888–901.

Bandelow B, Zohar J, Hollander E et al. World Federation of Societies of Biological Psychiatry (WFSBP) guidelines for the pharmacological treatment of anxiety, obsessive-compulsive and post-traumatic stress disorders – first revision. World J Biol Psychiatry 2008;9:248–312.

Barad M, Gean PW, Lutz B. The role of the amygdala in the extinction of conditioned fear. Biol Psychiatry 2006;60:322–8.

Becker CB, Zayfert C. Integrating DBT-Based techniques and concepts to facilitate exposure treatment for PTSD. Cogn Beh Prac 2001;8:107–22.

Berger W, Mendlowicz MV, Marques-Portella C et al. Pharmacologic alternatives to antidepressants in posttraumatic stress disorder: a systematic review. Prog Neuropsychopharmacol Biol Psychiatry 2009;33:169–80.

Binder EB, Bradley RG, Liu W et al. Association of FKBP5 polymorphisms and childhood abuse with risk of posttraumatic stress disorder symptoms in adults. JAMA 2008;299(11):1291–1305. [page 36]

Bisson J, Andrew M. Psychological treatment of post-traumatic stress disorder (PTSD). Cochrane Database Syst Rev 2007;3:CD003388.

Bliese PD, Wright KM, Adler AB et al. Validating the primary care posttraumatic stress disorder screen and the posttraumatic stress disorder checklist with soldiers returning from combat. J Consult Clin Psychol 2008;76(2):272–81.

Bouton ME, Westbrook RF, Corcoran KA, Maren S. Contextual and temporal modulation of extinction: behavioral and biological mechanisms. Biol Psychiatry 2006;60:352–60.

Bremner JD, Vythilingam M, Vermeten E et al. MRI and PET study of deficits in hippocampal structure and function in women with childhood sexual abuse and posttraumatic stress disorder. Am J Psychiatry 2003;160:92432.

Caspi A, Sugden K, Moffitt TE et al. Influence of life stress on depression: moderation by a polymorphism in the 5-HTT gene. Science 2003;301:386–9.

Charney DS. Psychobiological mechanisms of resilience and vulnerability: implications for successful adaptation to extreme stress. Am J Psychiatry 2004;161:195–216.

Connor KM, Foa DB, Davidson JRT. Practical assessment and evaluation of mental health problems following a mass disaster. J Clin Psychiatry 2006;67(suppl 2):26–33.

Corcoran KA, Quirk GJ. Recalling safety: cooperative functions of the ventromedial prefrontal cortex and the hippocampus in extinction. CNS Spectr 2005;10:820–30.

Czeh B, Muller-Keuker JIH, Rygula R et al. Chronic social stress inhibits cell proliferation in the adult medial prefrontal cortex: hemispheric asymmetry and reversal by fluoxetine treatment. Neuropsychopharmacol 2007;32:1490–1503.

Davis M, Ressler K, Rothbaum BO, Richardson R. Effects of d-cycloserine on extinction: translation from preclinical to clinical work. Biol Psychiatry 2006;60:369–75.

De Quervain DJ. Glucocorticoid-induced reduction of traumatic memories: implications for the treatment of PTSD. Prog Brain Res 2008;167:239–47.

De Quervain DJ, Aerni A, Roozendaal B. Preventive effect of beta adrenoceptor blockade on glucocorticoid-induced memory retrieval deficits. Am J Psychiatry 2007;164:967–9.

Engel Jr. CC, Liu X, McCarthy BD, Miller RF, Ursano R. Relationship of physical symptoms to posttraumatic stress disorder among veterans seeking care for Gulf war-related health concerns. Psychosom Med 2000;62:739–45. [page 161]

Eriksson PS, Wallin L. Functional consequences of stress-related suppression of adult hippocampal neurogenesis—a novel hypothesis on the neurobiology of burnout. Acta Neurol Scand 2004;110:275–80.

Fakra E, Hyde LW, Gorka A et al. Effects of HTR1A C(-1019)G on amygdala reactivity and trait anxiety. Arch Gen Psychiatry 2009;66(1):33–40.

Ferrari MCF, Busatto GF, McGuire PK, Crippa JAS. Structural magnetic resonance imaging in anxiety disorders: an update of research findings. Rev Bras Psiquiatr 2008;30(3):251–64.

Fox E, Ridgewell A, Ashwin C. Looking on the bright side: biased attention and the human serotonin transporter gene. Proc R Soc B 2009;276:1747–51.

Friedman MJ. Posttraumatic stress disorder among military returnees from Afghanistan and Iraq. Am J Psychiatry 2006;163(4):586–93.

Gilbertson MW, Shenton ME, Ciszewski A. Smaller hippocampal volume predicts pathologic vulnerability to psychological trauma. Nat Neurosci 2002;5(11):1242–7. [page 35]

Gross C, Hen R. The developmental origins of anxiety. Nat Neurosci 2004;5:545–52.

Hall RCW, Platt DE, Hall RCW. Suicide risk assessment: a review of risk factors for suicide in 100 patients who made severe suicide attempts. Psychosom 1999;40:18–27.

Hariri AR, Drabant EM, Weinberger DR. Imaging genetics: perspectives from studies of genetically driven variation in serotonin function and corticolimbic affective processing. Biol Psychiatry 2006;59:888–97.

Heim C, Nemeroff CB. Neurobiology of posttraumatic stress disorder. CNS Spectr 2009;14(suppl 1):13–24.

Hoge CW, Castro CA, Messer SC et al. Combat duty in Iraq and Afghanistan, mental health problems, and barriers to care. N Engl J Med 2004;351:13–22. [page 160]

Hoge CW, Auchterlonie JL, Milliken CS. Mental health problems, use of mental health services, and attrition from military service after returning from deployment to Iraq or Afghanistan. JAMA 2006;295(9):1023–32.

Hoge CW, Goldber HM, Castro CA. Care of war veterans with mild traumatic brain injury—flawed perspectives. N Engl J Med 2006;360:1588–81.

Hoge CW, McGurk D, Thomas JL et al. Mild traumatic brain injury in U.S. soldiers returning from Iraq. N Engl J Med 2008;358:453–63. [pages 167, 168]

Hoge CW, Terhakopian A, Castro CA, Messer SC, Engel CC. Association of posttraumatic stress disorder with somatic symptoms, health care visits, and absenteeism among Iraq war veterans. Am J Psychiatry 2007;164:150–3. [page 161]

Jeglic EL. Will my patient attempt suicide again? Cur Psychiatry 2008;7(11):19–31.

Karten YJG, Olariu A, Cameron HA. Stress in early life inhibits neurogenesis in adulthood. Trends Neurosci 2005;28:171–2.

Kasai K, Yamasue H, Gilbertson MW et al. Evidence for acquired pregenual anterior cingulate gray matter loss from a twin study of combat-related posttraumatic stress disorder. Biol Psychiatry 2008;63:550–6.

Kennedy JE, Jaffee MS, Leskin GA et al. Posttraumatic stress disorder and posttraumatic stress disorder-like symptoms and mild traumatic brain injury. J Regab Res Dev 2007;44:895–920.

Kessler RC, Sonnega A, Bromet E, Hughes M, Nelson CB. Posttraumatic stress disorder in the national comorbidity survey. Arch Gen Psychiatry 1995;52:1048–60. [pages 38, 39]

King NS. PTSD and traumatic brain injury: Folklore and fact? Brain Injury 2008;22:1–5.

Krystal AD, Davidson JRT. The use of prazosin for the treatment of trauma nightmares and sleep disturbance in combat veterans with posttraumatic stress disorder. Biol Psychiatry 2007;61:925–7.

Lanius RA, Bluhm R, Lanius U, Pain C. A review of neuroimaging studies in PTSD: heterogeneity of response to symptom provocation. J Psychiatric Res 2006;40:709–29.

Liedl S, O'Donnell M, Creamer M et al. Support for the mutual maintenance of pain and post-traumatic stress disorder symptoms. Psychol Med 2009; epub ahead of print. [page 40]

Lonsdorf TB, Weike AI, Nikamo P et al. Genetic gating of human fear learning and extinction. Psychological Sci 2009;20:198–206. [pages 45, 60]

Malberg JE, Duman RS. Cell proliferation in adult hippocampus is decreased by inescapable stress: reversal by fluoxetine treatment. Neuropsychopharmacol 2003;28:1562–71.

Mathew SJ, Price RB, Charney DS. Recent advances in the neurobiology of anxiety disorders: implications for novel therapeutics. Am J Med Genet C Semen Med Genet 2008;148C:89–98.

Miller L. Military psychology and police psychology: mutual contributions to crisis intervention and stress management. Int J Emerg Mental Health 2008;10:9–26.

Munafo MR, Brown SM, Hariri AR. Serotonin transporter (%-HTTLPR) genotype and amygdala activation: a meta-analysis. Biol Psychiatry 2008;63:852–7. [page 45]

Neigh GN, Gillespie CF, Nemeroff CB. The neurobiological toll of child abuse and neglect. Trauma Violence Abuse 2009;10:389–410.

Nock MK, Hwang I, Sampson NA, Kessler RC. Mental disorders, comorbidity and suicidal behavior: results from the National Comorbidity Survey Replication. Mol Psychiatry 2009;epub ahead of print. [page 31]

Nock MK, Hwang I, Sampson N et al. Cross-national analysis of the associations among mental disorders and suicidal behavior: findings from the WHO World Mental Health Surveys. PloS Med 2009;6(8):e1000123 epub ahead of print. [page 31]

North CS, Suris AM, Davis M, Smith RP. Toward validation of the diagnosis of posttraumatic stress disorder. Am J Psychiatry 2009;166:34–41.

Orr SP, Milad MR, Metzger LJ et al. Effects of beta blockade, PTSD diagnosis, and explicit threat on the extinction and retention of an aversively conditioned response. Biol Psychol 2006;732:262–71.

Otto MW, Basden SL, Leyro TM, McHugh K, Hofmann SG. Clinical perspectives on the combination of d-cycloserine and cognitive behavioral therapy for the treatment of anxiety disorders. CNS Spectr 2007;12:51-6, 59–61.

Panagioti M, Gooding P, Nicholas T. Post-traumatic stress disorder and suicidal behavior: a narrative review. Clin Psychology Rev 2009;29:471–82.

Parsey RV, Hastings RS, Oquendo MA et al. Effect of a triallelic functional polymorphism of the serotonin-transporter-linked promoter region on expression of serotonin transporter in the human brain. Am J Psychiatry 2006;163:48–51.

Paulus MP, Stein MB. An insular view of anxiety. Biol Psychiatry 2006;60:383–7.

Pezawas L, Meyer-Linden berg G, Drabant EM et al. 5-HTTLPR polymorphism impacts human cingulate-amygdala interactions: a genetic susceptibility mechanism for depression. Nat Neurosci 2005;8:828–34.

Phillips KA. Report of the DSM-V anxiety, obsessive-compulsive spectrum, posttraumatic, and dissociative disorders work group. http://psych.org/MainMenu/Research/DSMIV/DSMV/DSMRevisionActivities/DSMVWork GroupReports/AnxietyOCSpectrumPosttraumaticandDissociativeDisordersWorkGroupReport.aspx

Pitman RK, Sanders KM, Zusman RM et al. Pilot study of secondary prevention of post-traumatic stress disorder with propranolol. Biol Psychiatry 2002;51:189–92.

Quirk GJ, Garcia R, Gonzelez-Lima F. Prefrontal mechanisms in extinction of conditioned fear. Biol Psychiatgry 2006;60:337–42.

Raskind MA, Peskind ER, Hoff DJ et al. A parallel group placebo-controlled study of prazosin for trauma nightmares and sleep disturbance in combat veterans with post-traumatic stress disorder. Biol Psychiatry 2007;61:928–34.

Rasmussin AM, Pinna G, Paliwal P et al. Decreased cerebrospinal fluid allopregnanolone levels in women with PTSD. Biol Psychiatry 2006;60:704–13.

Rauch SL, Shin LM, Phelps EA. Neurocircuitry models of posttraumatic stress disorder and extinction: human neuroimaging research—past, present and future. Biol Psychiatry 2006;60:376–82.

Reist C, Duffy JG, Fujimoto K, Cahill L. Beta adrenergic blockade and emotional memory in PTSD. Int J Neuropsychopharmacol 2001;4:377–83.

Risch N, Herrel R, Lehner T et al. Interaction between the serotonin transporter gene (5-HTTLPR), stressful life events, and risk of depression: a meta-analysis. JAMA 2009;301:2462–71. [page 45]

Roberts NP, Kitchiner NJ, Kenardy J, Bisson J. Multiple session early psychological interventions for the prevention of post-traumatic stress disorder. Cochrane Database Syst Rev 2009;3:CD006869.

Rosen GM, Lilienfeld SO. Postraumatic stress disorder: an empirical evaluation of core assumptions. Clin Psychology Rev 2008;28:837–68.

Schelling G, Kilger E, Roozendaal B et al. Stress doses of hydrocortisone, traumatic memories, and symptoms of posttraumatic stress disorder in patients after cardiac surgery: a randomized study. Biol Psychiatry 2004;55:627–33.

Seal KH, Metzler TJ, Gima KA et al. Trends and risk factors for mental health diagnoses among Iraq and Afghanistant veterans using department of veterans affairs health care, 2002–2008. Am J Public Health 2009;99:1651–8. [page 165]

Shalev I, Lerer E, Israel S et al. BDNF val66met polymorphism is associated with HPA axis reactivity to psychological stress characterized by genotype and gender interactions. Psychoneuroendocrinol 2009;34:382–8.

Shin LM, Liberzon I. The neurocircuitry of fear, stress, and anxiety disorders. Neuropsychopharmacol 2009; epub ahead of print.

Spinelli S, Chefer S, Suomi SJ et al. Early-life stress induces long-term morphologic changes in primate brain. Arch Gen Psychiatry 2009;66:658–65.

Stahl SM. Stahl's essential psychopharmacology, third edition. New York, NY: Cambridge University Press; 2008.

Stahl SM. Stahl's illustrated chronic pain and fibromyalgia. New York, NY: Cambridge University Press; 2009.

Stein DJ, Ipser JC, Seedat S. Pharmacotherapy for post traumatic stress disorder (PTSD). Cochrane Database Syst Rev 2006;1:CD002795.

Stein MB, McAllister TW. Exploring the convergence of posttraumatic stress disorder and mild traumatic brain injury. Am J Psychiatry 2009;166:768–76.

Swanson CJ, Bures M, Johnson MP et al. Metabotropic glutamate receptors as novel targets for anxiety and stress disorders. Nat Rev 2005;4:131–44.

Vaiva G, Ducrocq F, Jezequel K et al. Immediate treatment with propranolol decreases posttraumatic stress disorder two months after trauma. Biol Psychiatry 2003;54:947–9.

Vermetten E, Vythilingam M, Southwick SM, Charney DS, Bremner JD. Long-term treatment with paroxetine increases verbal declarative memory and hippocampal volume in posttraumatic stress disorder. Biol Psychiatry 2003;54:693–702.

Whalen PJ, Kagan J, Cook RG et al. Human amygdala responsivity to masked fearful eye whites. Science 2004;306:2061.

Wittchen HU, Gloster A, Beesdo K, Schonfeld S, Perkonigg A. Posttraumatic stress disorder: diagnostic and epidemiological perspectives. CNS Spectr 2009;14(suppl 1):5–12.

Woon FL, Hedges DW. Hippocampal and amygdala volumes in children and adults with childhood maltreatment-related posttraumatic stress disorder: a meta-analysis. Hippocampus 2008;18:729–36. [page 35]

Zayfert C, Becker CB. Cognitive-behavioral therapy for PTSD: a case formulation approach. New York, NY: The Guilford Press; 2007.

*The information provided in Stahl's Illustrated Anxiety, Stress, and PTSD is an aggregate of all the references included here. References listed in orange text with page numbers are source publications for studies that are particularly highlighted within the text.

GABA-A receptors, 51, 102
GABA-B receptors, 51
gabapentin, 101, 153
GABA transaminase (GABA-T), 51
GABA transporter (GAT), 51
ganaxolone, 129
gender, and trauma types resulting in PTSD, 36, 37
generalized anxiety disorder: and alprazolam, 103; and duloxetine, 84; and escitalopram, 76
genetics: and risk factors for PTSD, 30, 34; and serotonin transporter gene, 42–3; and stress diathesis hypothesis, 19–22
Glasgow Coma Scale (GCS), 161, 164
glucocorticoid receptor antagonists, 128
glucocorticoids, 7, 8
glutamate, 40, 52–3
glycine, 53
gross stress reaction, 25
Gulf war, 160

headaches, and PTSD, 146
heart rate (HR), 6
hepatic impairment. See special populations
hippocampal atrophy: and chronic stress, 8, 33; and PTSD, 30–3, 35, 63
hippocampus: and beta blockers, 125; fear and fear conditioning, 11, 125; and inhibition of stress response, 8; and neuroimaging findings in PTSD, 35; small size of as risk factor in PTSD, 30. See also hippocampal atrophy
histamine 1 receptors, 92, 106
hydrocortisone, 124, 126
hyperarousal: and diagnostic criteria for PTSD, 26, 27; and exposure therapy, 133. See also arousal
hypertension: MAOIs and crisis of, 96; and prazosin, 110. See also blood pressure
hypnotics, and sedation, 109
hypocortisolism, 30

hypothalamic pituitary adrenal (HPA) axis: early life stress and dysregulation of, 31; and physiology of fear, 7; and PTSD, 31, 55, 128; and stress responses, 8, 54

iloperidone, 118
imaginal exposure, 133
imipramine, 93
impulse control, and suicide risk in PTSD, 29
infants, and exposure to stress, 18
information processing: and stress diathesis model, 20; and stress sensitized circuits, 17
insomnia: comorbidity of with PTSD, 152; and eszopiclone, 110; and tricyclic antidepressants, 92; and zaleplon, 110; and zolpidem, 110. See also sleep disturbances
interoceptive exposure, 133
investigational medications, 124
in vivo exposure, 133
Iraq war, 157–8, 160
irritability, and symptoms of PTSD, 27
irritable bowel syndrome, 146

kainate, 53

lamotrigine, 104, 120, 121, 148
locus coeruleus (LC): and noradrenergic projections, 46; and physiology of fear, 6
lorazepam, 103

magnetic resonance imaging (MRI), and traumatic brain injury, 161
MAOIs. See monoamine oxidase inhibitors
major depressive disorder: comorbidity of with PTSD, 28; and mirtazapine, 105; and neurophysiological alterations from early life stress, 31; and nortriptyline, 93; and selegiline, 99; and tranylcypromine, 99. See also depression

serotonin norepinephrine reuptake inhibitors (SNRIs): and chronic pain, 153; as first-line medications for PTSD, 60, 148; mechanisms of action, 78; and specific agents, 79

serotonin (5HT2C) receptors, and fluoxetine, 70

serotonin reuptake inhibition (SRI): and desvenlafaxine, 82; and duloxetine, 84; and escitalopram, 76; and fluoxetine, 70; and milnacipran, 86; and paroxetine, 66; and serotonin norepinephrine reuptake inhibitors, 78; and venlafaxine, 80. *See also* selective serotonin reuptake inhibitors (SSRIs)

serotonin syndrome, and MAOIs, 97

serotonin transporter (SERT): and citalopram, 74; and genetic risk factors for PTSD, 34; and genetics of amygdala response to fearful stimuli, 42–3; and mechanism of action of SSRIs, 61; and modulation of serotonergic neurotransmission, 44–5; and tricyclic antidepressants, 91

sertraline, 65, 68–9, 148

shell shock, 24

side effects: of citalopram, 75; of desvenlafaxine, 83; of duloxetine, 85; of escitalopram, 77; of fluoxetine, 71; of fluvoxamine, 73; of milnacipran, 87; of olanzapine, 113; of paroxetine, 67; of quetiapine, 114; of risperidone, 112; of sertraline, 69; of tricyclic antidepressants, 92; of venlafaxine, 81

sigma 1 receptors, 68, 72

SLC6A3 9 repeat allele, 34

sleep disturbances: and alpha 1 antagonists, 108; and diagnosis of PTSD, 27; and risperidone, 112; and sedative hypnotics, 109; treatment of PTSD and comorbid, 152. *See also* insomnia; nightmares

smoking cessation, 149

social support, and risk factors for PTSD, 30

sodium, and voltage-sensitive ion channels, 54

SPAN, 144

special populations: and citalopram, 75; and desvenlafaxine, 83; and duloxetine, 85; and escitalopram, 77; and fluoxetine, 71; and fluvoxamine, 73; and milnacipran, 87; and paroxetine, 67; and sertraline, 69; and venlafaxine, 81. *See also* infants; military population

startle responses, and diagnosis of PTSD, 27

stigma, as barrier to mental health care in military, 159

stimulants: and MAOIs, 97; and PTSD patients with postconcussive symptoms, 168

stress: exposure to in infancy, 18; and hippocampal volume, 33; and HPA activation, 7, 8; and neurobiology of sensitization to, 16–18; as risk factor for PTSD, 30, 31

stress diathesis model, 19–22

Stressful Life Events Screening Questionnaire (SLESQ), 144

stress inoculation training (SIT), 135, 136, 147

stroke, 7

substance abuse: comorbidity of with PTSD, 28, 149; and military populations, 156; and risk of suicide in PTSD, 29; and seeking safety therapy, 141. *See also* alcohol abuse

subsyndromal symptoms, 17

suicide and suicidal ideation: and military populations, 156, 157; risk of in PTSD patients, 29, 145

support groups, and comorbid PTSD and substance abuse, 149

temporomandibular joint disorders (TMJ), 160

threat with weapon, and risk of PTSD, 36, 37

To receive your certificate of CME credit or participation, please complete the posttest (you must score at least 70% to receive credit) and activity evaluation answer sheet found on the last page and return it by mail or fax it to 760-931-8713. Once received, your posttest will be graded and, along with your certificate (if a score of 70% or more was attained), returned to you by mail. Alternatively, <u>you may complete these items online and immediately print your certificate</u> at **www.neiglobal.com/cme**. There is a $40 fee for the posttest (waived for NEI members).

Please circle the correct answer on the answer sheet provided.

1. The emotional, physiological, and behavioral expressions of fear and anxiety are hypothetically regulated by circuitry centered around the:
   - A. Amygdala
   - B. Hippocampus
   - C. Hypothalamus
   - D. Prefrontal cortex

2. Individuals with PTSD demonstrate dysregulation of the HPA axis characterized by:
   - A. Increased CRF and glucocorticoids
   - B. Decreased CRF and glucocorticoids
   - C. Increased CRF and decreased glucocorticoids
   - D. Decreased CRF and increased glucocorticoids

3. Which of the following scenarios is consistent with the stress-diathesis model?
   - A. An individual with normal genes and an abusive childhood has inefficiently functioning brain circuits and a normal phenotype (i.e., no mental illness)
   - B. An individual with a risk gene and a normal childhood has inefficiently functioning brain circuits and a normal phenotype
   - C. An individual with both a risk gene and an abusive childhood has inefficiently function-ing brain circuits and a mental illness
   - D. A and C
   - E. A, B, and C

4. Although each first-line medication option for PTSD has a unique pharmacological profile, they all share what common central mechanism?
   - A. Dopamine reuptake inhibition
   - B. GABA reuptake inhibition
   - C. Serotonin reuptake inhibition
   - D. Norepinephrine reuptake inhibition

5. A 24-year-old male passenger suffers mild injuries in a head-on car accident in which the driver of the other vehicle dies. A beta blocker could theoretically be promising for individuals like this man because they have preliminarily been shown to:

A. Block formation of fear conditioning immediately following trauma

B. Reverse fear conditioning during exposure therapy

C. Facilitate fear extinction immediately following trauma

D. Facilitate fear extinction during exposure therapy

6. A man who was bitten by a dog as a child is beginning cognitive restructuring therapy to treat his PTSD. He identifies walking down the sidewalk past a person with their dog on a leash as a highly distressing situation, rating his fear during such an encounter as 80/100. He states that he strongly believes any dog is likely to escape its leash and try to attack him. The next step in cognitive restructuring would be for him to:

A. Put himself in a situation in which he encounters a dog on a leash

B. Identify evidence for and against the thought that the dog would escape and attack him

C. Practice techniques such as breathing exercises while thinking about encountering a dog on a leash

7. A young woman has just been diagnosed with PTSD and is ready to begin medication treatment. Which of the following has the most evidence of efficacy as a first-line treatment in PTSD?

A. Alprazolam

B. Duloxetine

C. Pregabalin

D. Sertraline

8. A patient presents with comorbid PTSD and substance abuse. Her care provider recommends seeking safety therapy as an initial treatment strategy prior to beginning any other CBT or medication. This means that:

A. PTSD will be addressed first

B. Substance abuse will be addressed first

C. PTSD and substance abuse will be addressed simultaneously

9. A 29-year-old woman has a history of childhood abuse and has suffered from depression and PTSD for many years without seeking treatment. She has just started taking a selective serotonin reuptake inhibitor. Based on general rates of remission with medications, symptoms of which disorder would be expected to improve the most?

A. Depression

B. PTSD

C. Depression and PTSD have comparable remission rates

10. A 22-year-old soldier has headaches, dizziness, irritability, and concentration problems six months after a blast injury in which he briefly lost consciousness. Both PTSD and persistent postconcussive syndrome are part of the differential diagnosis. According to existing data, which of these symptoms remains associated with brain injury after accounting for PTSD?

A. Headache

B. Dizzinesss

C. Irritability

D. Concentration problems

Stahl's Illustrated: Anxiety, Stress, and PTSD
Posttest and Activity Evaluation Answer Sheet

Please complete the posttest and activity evaluation answer sheet on this page and return by mail or fax. Alternatively, you may complete these items online and immediately print your certificate at **www.neiglobal.com/cme**. (Please circle the correct answer)

Posttest Answer Sheet (score of 70% or higher required for CME credit)

1.	A B C D	**6.**	A B C	
2.	A B C D	**7.**	A B C D	
3.	A B C D E	**8.**	A B C	
4.	A B C D	**9.**	A B C	
5.	A B C D	**10.**	A B C D	

Activity Evaluation: Please rate the following using a scale of: :

1-poor	2-below average	3-average	4-above average	5-excellent

1. The overall quality of the <u>content</u> was…
2. The overall quality of this <u>activity</u> was…   1 2 3 4 5
3. The relevance of the content to my professional needs was…   1 2 3 4 5
4. The level at which the learning objective was met of teaching me to explain the neurobiology of both normal and pathological stress and anxiety…   1 2 3 4 5
5. The level at which the learning objective was met of teaching me to recognize the environmental and genetic factors that can contribute to the development of anxiety disorders…   1 2 3 4 5
6. The level at which the learning objective was met of teaching me to explain the pharmacology of therapeutic agents used in treating posttraumatic stress disorder (PTSD)…   1 2 3 4 5
7. The level at which the learning objective was met of teaching me to identify new drugs and methods in development for the treatment of PTSD…   1 2 3 4 5
8. The level at which the learning objective was met of teaching me to explain the principles and methods involved in cognitive behavioral therapy (CBT) for PTSD…   1 2 3 4 5
9. The level at which the learning objective was met of teaching me to customize treatment regimens for patients with PTSD based on symptom profile, comorbidities, and life situations…   1 2 3 4 5
10. The level at which this activity was objective, scientifically balanced, and free of commercial bias was…   1 2 3 4 5
11. Based on my experience and knowledge, the level of this activity was…   1 2 3 4 5
    Too Basic   Basic   Appropriate   Complex   Too Complex
12. My confidence level in understanding and treating this topic has _____ as a result of participating in this activity.
    A.   Increased   B.   Stayed the same   C.   Decreased

13. Based on the information presented in this activity, I will…
    A.   Change my practice   C.   Do nothing as current practice reflects activity's recommendations
    B.   Seek additional information on this topic   D.   Do nothing as the content was not convincing

(continued on next page)

14. I commit to making the following change(s) in my practice as a result of participating in this activity.
    A. Educate PTSD patients and their families on PTSD, its neurobiological and environmental contributors, and the scientific rationale for various treatment options
    B. Encourage patients with PTSD to participate in cognitive behavioral therapy
    C. Assess for comorbidities and complications prior to making treatment recommendations as well as periodically during treatment
    D. A and B
    E. A and C
    F. B and C
    G. All of the changes (A, B, and C)
    H. I am already doing all of the above

15. What barriers might keep you from implementing changes in your practice you'd like to make as a result of participating in this activity?

16. The following additional information about this topic would help me in my practice:

17. How could this activity have been improved?

Number of credits I am claiming, commensurate with the extent of my participation in the activity (maximum of 4.0): _____

Name: _____ Creditentials: _____

Address: _____

City, State, Zip: _____

Email: _____ Phone: _____

Method of Payment: Check   Visa   Mastercard   NEI Member #: _____

Credit Card #: _____ Exp. Date: _____

Signature: _____ Date: _____

Amount Authorized: $40.00

Mail or fax <u>both sides</u> of this form to:

Mail: CME Department   Fax: 760-931-8713
         Neuroscience Education Institute   Attn: CME Department
         1930 Palomar Point Way, Suite 101
         Carlsbad, CA 92008